Respiratory Disease Series: Diagnostic Tools and Disease Managements

Series Editors
Hiroyuki Nakamura
Ibaraki Medical Center
Tokyo Medical University
Ibaraki, Japan

Kazutetsu Aoshiba
Ibaraki Medical Center
Tokyo Medical University
Ibaraki, Japan

This book series cover a variety of topics in respiratory diseases, with each volume providing an overview of the current state of knowledge, recent discoveries and future prospects for each disease. In each chapter the editors pose critical questions, which are often unresolved clinical issues. These are then discussed by the authors, providing insights and suggestions as to which developments need to be addressed. The series offers new information, which will inspire innovative ideas to further develop respiratory medicine.This collection of monographs is aimed at benefiting patients across the globe suffering from respiratory disease.

Edited by established authorities in the field and written by pioneering experts, this book series will be valuable to those researchers and physicians working in respiratory medicine. The series is aimed at a broad readership, and the books will also be a valuable resource for radiologists, emergency medicine physicians, pathologists, pharmacologists and basic research scientists.

More information about this series at http://www.springer.com/series/15152

Akihito Yokoyama
Editor

Advances in Asthma

Pathophysiology, Diagnosis and Treatment

Springer

Editor
Akihito Yokoyama
Department of Hematology and Respiratory Medicine
Kochi Medical School
Nankoku-shi
Kochi
Japan

ISSN 2509-5552 ISSN 2509-5560 (electronic)
Respiratory Disease Series: Diagnostic Tools and Disease Managements
ISBN 978-981-13-2789-6 ISBN 978-981-13-2790-2 (eBook)
https://doi.org/10.1007/978-981-13-2790-2

Library of Congress Control Number: 2018964247

This Springer imprint is published by the registered company Springer Nature Singapore Pte Ltd.
The registered company address is: 152 Beach Road, #21-01/04 Gateway East, Singapore 189721, Singapore

Preface

Bronchial asthma is one of the common diseases among the Japanese, accounting for about 6–10% of the population. A rising prevalence of allergic diseases, such as asthma, had been observed in the past 20–30 years and had been attributed to both Western lifestyle and fewer infections. However, this prevalence has started to decline somewhat in recent years.

The effectiveness of inhaled corticosteroids (ICS) became clear since the 1980s. This led to the recognition that airway inflammation, particularly the eosinophilic type, is an essential characteristic of asthma. There is no doubt that the guidelines for asthma have greatly contributed to the spread of ICS use in various countries, including Japan. At the same time, understanding of the mechanism of eosinophilic asthma has greatly improved, owing to both the discovery of functional dichotomy (i.e., Th1, Th2) of the CD4-positive T cell clones and the development of the mouse asthma model. The schema of asthma that was equated to eosinophilic airway inflammation was emphasized in those days.

On the other hand, in the late 1990s, the existence of non-eosinophilic asthma was demonstrated, and it became clear that asthma cannot be regarded as a single disease. At present, examination of induced sputum revealed that airway inflammation is divided into 4 types, including eosinophilic, neutrophilic, mixed, and paucigranulocytic. When considering the treatment of more severe asthma, the phenotypes and endotypes reflecting the underlying mechanism of asthmatic airway inflammation should be considered. Furthermore, it is now clear that innate lymphoid cells (ILCs) have important roles in airway inflammation. In particular, involvement of ILC2 in ICS-resistant eosinophilic inflammation and ILC3 in neutrophilic airway inflammation in obesity had been reported.

In this volume of the respiratory disease series, we summarized the progress of basic science, such as the genetics and immunology mentioned above, followed by several issues on diagnosis, including phenotype and endotype, periostin, exhaled nitric oxide (FeNO), forced oscillation technique, and aspirin-exacerbated asthma. Furthermore, we described the recent progress in treatment, such as the renewed guidelines for asthma, knowledge and guidance on the use of asthma inhalers, bronchial thermoplasty, asthma-COPD overlap, and the current and future biologics, such as anti-IgE antibody and anti-IL-4α receptor antibody for severe asthma.

These topics will provide the physicians with a comprehensive appreciation of the mechanisms, pathophysiology, diagnosis, and treatment of bronchial asthma. There are some differences between the Western and Asian populations in terms of the diagnosis and treatment of asthma, and sharing this experience on a Japanese population may be beneficial for clinicians in Asia. Therefore, this book may come in handy and useful for clinical application and patient care. Moreover, the information in this book could stimulate asthma research in the future. Finally, I appreciate the enthusiastic participation of all the contributors who prepared the outstanding state-of-the-art reviews.

Kochi, Japan Akihito Yokoyama

Contents

Part III Treatment

Part I
Pathophysiology

Chapter 1
Genetics in Asthma

Tohru Sakamoto and Nobuyuki Hizawa

Abstract Asthma is a complex disease determined by the interaction between genetic and environmental factors. The heritability of asthma is estimated to be more than 50%. The search for genes with genomic variants associated with asthma has been greatly advanced by hypothesis-driven candidate gene association studies and hypothesis-free genome-wide association studies (GWASs). The genes identified by the hypothesis-driven approach are roughly classified into four types of functional group: (1) innate immunity and immunoregulation, (2) differentiation and regulation of T-helper 2 cells, (3) airway epithelial mucosal immunity, and (4) airway remodeling and lung function. Although the majority of the variants have been identified by the hypothesis-driven approach, novel genes and pathways associated with asthma have been successively clarified by GWASs. Nonetheless, these genomic variants explain only a small proportion of asthma heritability. This is partly due to the phenotypic heterogeneity of asthma, epistatic gene-gene interactions, gene-environment interactions, and epigenetic effects. Further elucidation of the causal variants can be achieved by GWASs that limit participants to those with distinct asthma phenotypes and by integrative applications of genome-wide epistatic and epigenetic approaches. Understanding of the genetic profiles of asthma pathogenesis contributes to individualized disease prevention as well as to development of new therapies.

Keywords Association study · Epigenetics · Epistasis · Gene-environment interaction

T. Sakamoto (✉) · N. Hizawa
Department of Pulmonary Medicine, Faculty of Medicine, University of Tsukuba, Tsukuba, Japan
e-mail: t-saka@md.tsukuba.ac.jp

A. Yokoyama (ed.), *Advances in Asthma*, Respiratory Disease Series: Diagnostic Tools and Disease Managements, https://doi.org/10.1007/978-981-13-2790-2_1

1.1 Introduction

Asthma is a complex syndrome characterized by reversible airflow obstruction, airway hyperresponsiveness, and chronic airway inflammation. Although asthma has been recognized as a disease with heritable components, the increase in asthma prevalence, especially in developed countries, suggests that both genetic and environmental factors are involved in its pathogenesis. The different clinical phenotypes of asthma also reflect a variety of interactions between multiple genetic and environmental risk factors. In regard to the genetic contribution, a recent meta-analysis of 71 twin studies estimated the heritability of asthma to be 54% [1]. In the past few decades, the search for genes associated with asthma has been rigorously carried out, and almost 700 genes have been reported. A major breakthrough in this identification of the genes has been achieved by genetic association studies, i.e., candidate gene and genome-wide association (GWAS) studies. Although more than half of the identified genes have not been replicated by other studies, the numerous remaining genes with repeated validations confirm that the disease risk depends on many different genetic variants. Characterizing the genetic architecture of asthma contributes to understanding of its pathophysiological mechanisms and leads to the discovery of new biological drugs. The genetic profiles associated with asthma susceptibility are extremely useful for identifying at-risk individuals and for performing early intervention. And the genetic profiling for progression, severity, and therapeutic response of asthma can significantly contribute to modifying the disease's progression, preventing severe disease, and developing personalized medicine.

In this chapter, we first summarize the results of association studies on asthma and discuss their limitations. We then discuss the genetic approaches to asthma pathogenesis considering the presence of disease heterogeneity, epistasis (gene-gene interactions), gene-environment (GxE) interactions, and epigenetics.

1.2 Association Studies

Genetic association studies test for relationships between disease traits and genetic variations such as single-nucleotide polymorphisms (SNPs) to identify candidate genes for the disease. Such studies usually compare the allele or genotype frequencies of individuals with the disease and healthy controls (case-control association study). Genetic association studies can be further differentiated into two approaches: hypothesis-driven candidate gene association studies and hypothesis-free GWASs.

1.2.1 Candidate Gene Association Studies

In candidate gene association studies, genes are generally selected on the basis of their known function that is hypothesized to influence asthma susceptibility or on the basis of their chromosomal position identified by previous linkage studies. Although associations identified by this method are easy to interpret, candidate gene association studies cannot discover novel genes or pathways. To validate an association, the association must be replicated in at least several independent studies. According to the DisGeNET database [2], almost 700 genes associated with asthma have been reported as a result of using this method, and around 100 genes have been replicated more than 4 times at the gene level. The gene level means that any variants associated with asthma are considered to represent a replication if they are located within the same gene. Figure 1.1 provides a summary of the top 30 genes identified first by candidate gene association studies and subsequently replicated in at least 15 independent reports. These genes are classified into four functional categories [3], as described hereafter:

(1) Genes associated with innate immunity and immunoregulation: Pattern-recognition receptors such as CD14 and TLR4 can be triggered by a variety of environmental stimuli, which leads to secretion of mediators stimulating adaptive immune responses. CTLA4, TGFB1, IL10, and IFNG are immunoregulatory cytokines. CTLA4 contributes to the suppressor function of regulatory T cells; thus, dysregulation of CTLA4 has the potential to affect the pathogenesis of asthma. TGFB1 has profound immunosuppressive actions involving both innate and adaptive responses. IL10 regulates the immune response by inhibiting antigen-presenting cells. IFNG is important for the activation of macrophages. By upregulating Th1 responses, IFNG subsequently inhibits Th2 differentiation. Each of these immunoregulatory cytokines plays an important role in orchestrating both innate and adaptive immunity. HLA class II molecules such as HLA-DRB1 and HLA-DQB1 are essential for activation of antigen-specific T cells.
(2) Genes associated with differentiation and regulation of Th2 cells: IL4, IL13, and their receptor, IL4R, are critically involved in the onset and effector phase of Th2 immune responses. MS4A2, also known as FCER1B, is a high-affinity IgE receptor and stimulates Th2 responses. Conversely, IL12B induces differentiation of Th1 cells and downregulates Th2 responses.
(3) Genes expressed in epithelial cells and involved in mucosal immunity: CCL5, also known as RANTES, is a chemoattractant for Th cells and eosinophils. SCGBA1 is a clara cell secretory protein and plays an important role in immunoregulation. FLG, an essential regulator of epidermal homeostasis, is highly associated with atopic dermatitis and influences susceptibility to asthma. Interestingly, FLG is not expressed in bronchial epithelial cells, which led to the concept of the atopic march.
(4) Genes associated with airway remodeling and lung function: This category includes genes related to inflammatory responses (*TNF*, *LTC4S*, *LTA*, *ALOX5*, *IL18*, *ACE*, *IL1RN*, *CCR5*, and *IL6*), detoxification (*GSTP1*, *GSTM1*, and *GSTT1*), and bronchoconstriction (*ADRB2* and *CYSLTR1*). TGFB1 is the master regulator of fibrosis [4] and acts as an immunoregulatory cytokine.

Gene	Chromosome	Function
ADRB2	5q32	Bronchial smooth-muscle relaxation
TNF	6p21.33	Inflammatory responses
IL13	5q31.1	Th2-cell differentiation and effector functions
IL4	5q31.1	Th2-cell differentiation and effector functions
IL4R	16p12.1	Th2-cell differentiation and effector functions
GSTP1	11q13.2	Environmental and oxidative stress — detoxification
GSTM1	1p13.3	Environmental and oxidative stress — detoxification
CD14	5q31.3	Innate immunity — microbial recognition
TGFB1	19q13.2	Immunoregulation, profibrotic effects
CCL5	17q12	Monocyte, T-cell, and eosinophil chemoattractant
LTC4S	5q35.3	Inflammatory responses
IL10	1q32.1	Immunoregulation
MS4A2	11q12.1	Th2-cell differentiation and effector functions
SCGB1A1	11q12.3	Epithelium-derived anti-inflammatory responses
TLR4	9q33.1	Innate immunity and immunoregulation
GSTT1	22q11.23	Environmental and oxidative stress — detoxification
FLG	1q21.3	Epithelial barrier integrity
LTA	6p21.33	Inflammatory responses
CYSLTR1	Xq21.1	Bronchoconstriction
HLA-DRB1	6p21.32	Antigen presentation
ALOX5	10q11.21	Inflammatory and allergic responses
HLA-DQB1	6p21.32	Antigen presentation
IL18	11q23.1	Inflammatory responses
ACE	17q23.3	Inhibition of inflammatory responses
IFNG	12q15	Innate and adaptive immune responses
CTLA4	2q33.2	T-cell-response inhibition and immunoregulation
IL12B	5q33.3	Downregulation of Th2 responses
IL1RN	2q14.1	Inhibition of inflammatory responses
CCR5	3p21.31	Inflammatory responses to infection
IL6	7p15.3	Inflammatory responses

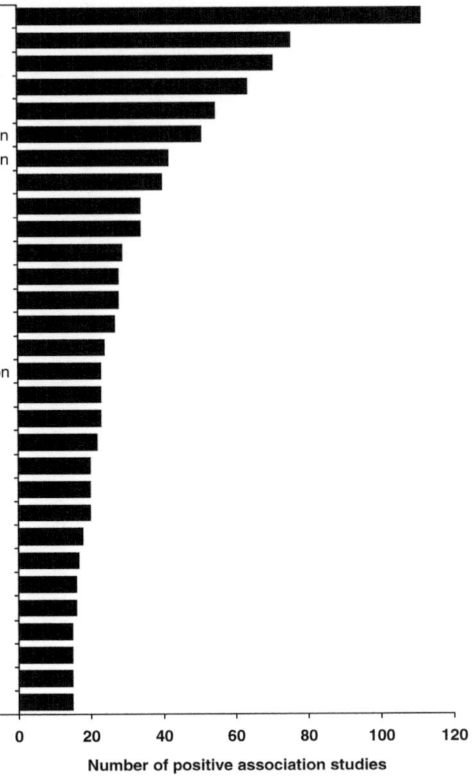

Fig. 1.1 Top 30 genes identified by candidate gene association studies on asthma. Genes associated with asthma in at least 15 independent reports were selected by searching the public database DisGeNET (http://www.disgenet.org/web/DisGeNET/menu;jsessionid=1fhetotkci0swxh27imgj7tdg). *ADAM33* and *NPSR1* were excluded because associations of these two genes with asthma were first reported by hypothesis-free linkage analysis followed by positional cloning

Although associations of *ADAM33* and *NPSR1* with asthma have been replicated in 27 and 16 independent candidate gene association studies, respectively, we have excluded these two genes from Fig. 1.1 because associations of the genes with asthma were first reported by hypothesis-free linkage analysis followed by positional cloning. ADAM 33 is preferentially expressed in mesenchymal cells such as smooth muscle cells and fibroblasts, but not in bronchial epithelium and inflammatory cells. This membrane-anchored protein is implicated in a variety of biological processes involving cell-cell and cell-matrix interactions. It is suggested that ADAM33 is a tissue remodeling protein and affects airflow obstruction and lung function [5]. The identification of ADAM33 provided an important breakthrough in understanding epithelial-mesenchymal interactions in the pathogenesis of asthma. NPSR1 is a G protein-coupled receptor for neuropeptide S and related to multiple neuroendocrine and inflammatory responses. NPSR1 is highly expressed in the bronchial epithelium and smooth muscle cells of asthma patients.

1.2.2 Genome-Wide Association Studies

GWAS allows the analysis of hundreds of thousands to millions of polymorphisms located throughout the genome and permits unbiased or hypothesis-free study. Table 1.1 shows a summary of GWASs on asthma from the GWAS Catalogue (https://www.ebi.ac.uk/gwas/). To date, 17 GWASs on asthma identified 83 SNPs with a standard genome-wide significance level ($P < 5 \times 10^{-8}$) in the discovery data.

The first asthma-associated locus identified by GWAS is located on chromosome 17q21, which includes the *ORMDL3* and *GSDMB* genes [6]. The function of ORMDL3 and GSDMB in asthma had been largely unknown. However, after this first GWAS, associations of *ORMDL3* and *GSDMB* with asthma were replicated in 17 and 16 independent candidate gene association studies, respectively. The SNPs identified by these studies are strongly associated with increased expression of both *ORMDL3* and *GSDMB* [7]. Recently, it has been shown that intrinsically elevated levels of ORMDL3 in the endoplasmic reticulum of airway smooth muscle cells upregulate their own contractility and proliferation, which might contribute to airway hyperresponsiveness (AHR) independent of extrinsic inflammation [8]. GSDMB is highly expressed in human bronchial epithelial cells in asthma. Overexpression of GSDMB increases expression of 5-lipoxygenase and TGFB1 in bronchial epithelium, which also leads to AHR and airway remodeling in the absence of inflammation [9]. The understanding of these functions of both ORMDL3 and GSDMB challenges the current paradigm that AHR and airway remodeling in asthma are secondary to airway inflammation.

Another promising GWAS locus for asthma is *IL33* on chromosome 9q24, which has been replicated in six independent asthma GWASs. IL33 is an innate epithelial cytokine and released from inflamed or injured epithelial cells. *IL1RL1*, on chromosome 2q12, encoding part of the IL33 receptor complex, has also been replicated in five asthma GWASs. IL1RL1 is expressed on Th2 cells, type 2 innate lymphoid

Table 1.1 Summary of genome-wide association studies on asthma ($P < 5 \times 10^{-8}$)

First author	Journal	Disease/ trait	Ethnicity	SNP	Gene	*P* value
Moffatt MF	Nature, 2007	Childhood asthma	European	rs7216389	*ORMDL3*	9×10^{-11}
Himes BE	Am J Hum Genet, 2009	Childhood asthma	European	rs1588265	*PDE4D*	3×10^{-8}
Sleiman PM	N Engl J Med, 2010	Childhood asthma	European	rs2786098	*DENND1B–CRB1*	9×10^{-11}
Moffatt MF	N Engl J Med, 2010	Asthma	European	rs3771166 rs744910 rs3894194 rs2284033 rs9273349 rs1342326	*IL18R1* *SMAD3* *GSDMA* *IL2RB* *HLA-DQA1–* *HLA-DQB1* *IL33*	3×10^{-9} 4×10^{-9} 5×10^{-9} 1×10^{-8} 7×10^{-14} 9×10^{-10}
Torgerson DG	Nat Genet, 2011	Asthma	European African Latino	rs1101999 rs3771180 rs1837253 rs2381416 rs11078927	*PYHIN1* (African) *IL1RL1* *TSLP* *IL33* *GSDMB*	4×10^{-9} 2×10^{-15} 1×10^{-14} 2×10^{-12} 2×10^{-16}
Hirota T	Nat Genet, 2011	Asthma	Japanese	rs7686660 rs1837253 rs204993 rs404860 rs3129943 rs3117098 rs3129890 rs7775228 rs9275698 rs9500927 rs10508372 rs2069408 rs1701704	*LOC729675* *TSLP* *PBX2* *NOTCH4* *C6orf10* *BTNL2* *HLA-DRA* *HLA-DQB1* *HLA-DQA2* *HLA-DOA* *LOC338591* *CDK2* *IKZF4*	2×10^{-12} 1×10^{-16} 2×10^{-15} 4×10^{-23} 3×10^{-15} 5×10^{-12} 5×10^{-13} 5×10^{-15} 5×10^{-12} 4×10^{-9} 2×10^{-15} 1×10^{-10} 2×10^{-13}
Noguchi E	PLoS Genet, 2011	Childhood asthma	Japanese	rs3019885 rs987870	*SLC30A8* *HLA-DPB1*	5×10^{-13} 2×10^{-10}
Ferreira MA	Lancet, 2011	Asthma	European	rs4129267 rs7130588	*IL6R* *LRRC32*	2×10^{-8} 2×10^{-8}
Forno E	J Allergy Clin Immunol, 2012	Childhood asthma	European	rs9815663 rs7927044	*IL5RA* *NR*	2×10^{-8} 7×10^{-9}
Wan YI	Thorax, 2012	Asthma	European	rs4794820	*ORMDL3*	1×10^{-8}
Ramasamy A	PLoS One, 2012	Asthma	European	rs13408661 rs9268516	*IL18R1–* *IL1RL1* *HLA-DRA–* *BTNL2*	1×10^{-9} 1×10^{-8}
Lasky-Su J	Clin Exp Allergy, 2012	Asthma	European	rs9272346	*HLA-DQA1*	2×10^{-8}
Ding L	Hum Genomics, 2013	Childhood asthma	European African Hispanic	rs16929097 rs17218161 rs12570188	Intergenic Intergenic *HPSE2*	8×10^{-9} 2×10^{-8} 5×10^{-8}

Table 1.1 (continued)

First author	Journal	Disease/ trait	Ethnicity	SNP	Gene	*P* value
Bonnelykke K	Nat Genet, 2013	Childhood asthma	European	rs6967330	*CDHR3*	3×10^{-14}
				rs2305480	*GSDMB*	6×10^{-23}
				rs928413	*IL33*	9×10^{-13}
				rs3894194	*GSDMA*	3×10^{-21}
Ferreira MA	J Allergy Clin Immunol, 2013	Asthma and hay fever	European	rs9273373	*HLA-DQB1*	4×10^{-14}
				rs4833095	*TLR1*	5×10^{-12}
				rs1438673	*WDR36*	3×10^{-11}
				rs10197862	*IL1RL1*	4×10^{-11}
				rs7212938	*GSDMA*	4×10^{-10}
				rs1837253	*TSLP*	1×10^{-9}
				rs72699186	*IL33*	2×10^{-9}
				rs17294280	*SMAD3*	4×10^{-9}
				rs7009110	*ZBTB10*	4×10^{-9}
				rs62026376	*CLEC16A*	1×10^{-8}
Pickrell JK	Nat Genet, 2016	Asthma	European	rs11655198	*ZPBP2*	1×10^{-63}
				rs3104367	*HLA-DRB5–*	1×10^{-40}
				rs144829310	*HLA-DQA1*	1×10^{-31}
				rs1837253	*RANBP6–*	3×10^{-31}
				rs202011557	*IL33*	5×10^{-31}
				rs56375023	*SLC25A46–*	2×10^{-21}
				rs7936323	*TSLP*	1×10^{-16}
				rs2428494	*IL1RL2–*	1×10^{-16}
				rs2244012	*IL1RL1*	2×10^{-16}
				rs34290285	*SMAD3*	2×10^{-15}
				rs7203459	*C11orf30–*	4×10^{-15}
				rs4233366	*LRRC32*	5×10^{-15}
				rs12413578	*HLA-C–MICA*	8×10^{-12}
				rs10957978	*RAD50*	1×10^{-11}
				rs10519068	*D2HGDH*	4×10^{-11}
				rs5743618	*CLEC16A*	4×10^{-11}
				rs58521088	*B4GALT3–*	7×10^{-11}
				rs3001426	*ADAMTS4*	1×10^{-10}
				rs73196739	*GATA3*	7×10^{-9}
				rs6683383	*TPD52–*	1×10^{-8}
				rs13412757	*ZBTB10*	1×10^{-8}
				rs1723018	*RORA*	1×10^{-8}
				rs3784099	*TLR1*	2×10^{-8}
				rs6959584	*BACH2*	2×10^{-8}
				rs200634877	*STAT6–LRP1*	3×10^{-8}
				rs6691738	*LPP*	3×10^{-8}
				rs662064	*ADORA1*	3×10^{-8}
					ID2	
					CD247	
					RAD51B	
					CDHR3	
					NDFIP1	
					TNFSF18–	
					TNFSF4	
					PEX14	

(continued)

Table 1.1 (continued)

First author	Journal	Disease/ trait	Ethnicity	SNP	Gene	*P* value
Almoguera B	Am J Respir Crit Care Med, 2017	Asthma Adult asthma	African European	rs11788591 rs72721168 rs1776883 rs75446656 rs36080042 rs3095318	*PTGES* *MOB3B–EQTN–TEK* *GRM4–HGMA1* *JMJD1C* *REEP3* *PSORS1C1*	4×10^{-8} 7×10^{-10} 5×10^{-9} 4×10^{-8} 5×10^{-8} 2×10^{-11}

cells (ILC2s), and innate immune cells such as mast cells and basophils. The IL33/IL1RL1 signaling pathway induces type 2 immune responses. These findings emphasize an important role of innate epithelial cytokines in promoting type 2 immune responses related to asthma pathogenesis. TSLP is also an innate epithelial cytokine, which has been replicated in five independent asthma GWASs. TSLP is released in response to environmental stimuli and induces type 2 immune responses by activating dendritic cells, ILC2s, and T cells. TLR1 also plays an important role in regulation of adaptive as well as innate immune responses. TLR1 forms a heterodimer with TLR2 and recognizes a wide variety of microbial ligands. Association of *TLR1* with asthma has been replicated in three independent GWASs.

As predicted by their function in activation of antigen-specific T cells, associations of HLA class II molecule genes (*HLA-DQ*, *HLA-DR*, *HLA-DP*, and *HLA-DO*) with asthma have been replicated in several independent GWASs.

Recently, a large GWAS involving 28,399 asthma cases and 128,843 controls demonstrated 27 SNPs, with a significance of $P < 5 \times 10^{-8}$ [10]. Six of these SNPs showed *P* values even lower than 1×10^{-20}. Each of these six SNPs is located in the locus containing *ZPBP2* ($P = 1.0 \times 10^{-63}$), *HLA-DRB5–HLA-DQA1* ($P = 1 \times 10^{-40}$), *RANBP6–IL33* ($P = 1.3 \times 10^{-31}$), *SLC25A46–TSLP* ($P = 3.3 \times 10^{-31}$), *IL1RL2–IL1RL1* ($P = 5.1 \times 10^{-31}$), and *SMAD3* ($P = 2.4 \times 10^{-21}$). The *ZPBP2* gene is located in a dense haploblock on chromosome 17q21 encompassing the *ORMDL3*, *GSDMB*, *GSDMA*, and *IKZF3* genes. Asthma-risk alleles in this locus affect the expression of *ORMDL3* and *GSDMB* [7], which may lead to AHR and airway remodeling. *HLA-DRB5* and *HLA-DQA1* are HLA class II genes responsible for adaptive immune responses. As mentioned above, TSLP and IL1RL1 play an important role in linking innate and adaptive immunity in asthma, and both have been replicated in several independent asthma GWASs. SMAD3 is a downstream mediator of TGFB1 and plays a central role in regulating airway smooth muscle cell proliferation and airway remodeling [11]. SMAD3 has been replicated in four independent asthma GWASs.

Although GWASs have identified many previously unknown candidate genes, which have led in turn to understanding of novel biological mechanisms and pathways of asthma susceptibility, the genetic variants identified so far explain only a small proportion of the heritability. This is partly due to the fact that GWAS deals primarily with common variants with minor allele frequencies >1%. Rare variants and structure variants (duplications, inversions, translocations, and copy-number repeats) that are not included in available genotyping arrays might play an important role in the pathogenesis of common diseases such as asthma. Other potential reasons stem from the phenotypic heterogeneity of asthma, epistasis (gene-gene interactions), GxE interactions, and epigenetic effects. Despite these limitations, GWASs have still given rise to many novel concepts related to the pathogenesis of asthma.

1.3 Phenotypic Heterogeneity, Epistasis, Gene-Environment Interactions, and Epigenetics

Unbiased cluster analyses have demonstrated that asthma is a syndrome with heterogeneous phenotypic groups [12]. To increase the statistical power to detect true variants associated with asthma, several recent GWASs focused on distinct asthma phenotypes. We identified the *HCG22* gene through a GWAS focusing on late-onset asthma (age of onset ≥40 years) [13]. And a GWAS limiting participants to those with a smoking history of no more than 10 pack-years identified *HAS2* as a susceptibility gene for adult asthma [14].

Epistasis is defined as the interaction between two or more genes affecting a phenotype of interest. The combined effect of multiple loci on the phenotype is not additive but rather synergistic or antagonistic. Several epistatic effects on asthma have been studied by focusing on interactions between *IL4*- and *IL13*-related genes [15]. Other epistatic effects on asthma include interactions between innate immunity-related genes such as *CD14* and *AOAH* [16], between oxidative stress-related genes such as *NQO1*, *MPO*, and *CAT* [17], and between airway remodeling-related genes such as *PAI-1* and *MS4A2* [18]. These studies have used candidate gene approaches for analysis of the epistatic interactions. Hypothesis-free analysis of genome-wide epistatic interactions is severely hampered by a huge number of SNP-SNP combinations, which leads to significant difficulties in attaining sufficient statistical power. When all possible pairs of genes in a GWAS including 500,000 SNPs are selected, potentially 250 billion interactions must be tested. Nevertheless, several statistical methods have been developed to identify genome-wide epistatic interactions. Recently, an epistatic interaction between *ADAM33* and *GLI2* has been reported as a result of a genome-wide search [19]. As the transcriptional factor GLI2 regulates TGFB1 expression in $CD4^+$ T cells [20], GLI2 also seems to be involved in the pathogenesis of asthma.

GxE interactions are another possible reason for why the identified genetic variants explain only a small proportion of the heritability. Although the GxE interactions in asthma have been well recognized, the necessity for a large number of samples and the difficulties in accurately assessing environmental exposures mean that only a few comprehensive studies have been performed to date. The results of the genome-wide GxE interaction studies of asthma have been disappointing, with none of them meeting genome-wide criteria for statistical significance. The majority of the GxE interaction studies dealt with candidate GxE interactions, especially interactions between microbial exposures and variants in genes of the innate and adaptive immune systems and between oxidant exposures and variants in antioxidant genes. Interaction between endotoxin exposure and a variant in endotoxin signaling pathway genes including *CD14* is associated with asthma susceptibility [21]. Interactions between oxidant air pollutants and antioxidant genes such as *CAT* and *HMOX-1* contribute to asthma susceptibility during adolescence [22].

GxE interactions can also be mediated by epigenetic modifications of the genome. Epigenetic modifications are caused by environmental stimuli and are defined as heritable changes in gene expression that do not involve changes in the underlying DNA sequence. Three types of genetic modifications are recognized to cause epigenetic effects: DNA methylation, histone modification, and noncoding RNA-associated gene silencing. Among these modifications, DNA methylation has been extensively focused on because a quantitative survey of methylation modification has recently become widely available. DNA methylation is covalent binding of a methyl group to the cytosine ring of genomic DNA. In humans, DNA methylation typically occurs at a cytosine nucleotide adjacent to a guanine residue (CpG dinucleotide) in somatic cells. Hypermethylation in the promoter region of the gene leads to gene silencing, while hypomethylation leads to active transcription. The effects of methylation in intragenic regions are complex and less clear. The majority of DNA methylation studies use genomic DNA isolated from leukocytes or mononuclear cells because these cells are readily collected from blood. Several array-based platforms for genome-wide methylation analysis are now available.

A genome-wide methylation study with blood mononuclear cells of inner-city children identified 81 differentially methylated regions in asthma patients when compared with healthy controls [23]. Several immunity-related genes involved in T cell maturation (*RUNX3*), Th2 immune responses (*IL13, IL4* and *TIGIT*), and oxidative stress (*CAT*) were hypomethylated in the asthmatic patients. Considering the functions of these genes, the results seem to be reasonable. However, whether the differentially methylated regions are causes or consequences of asthma development is difficult to determine. Methylation studies with blood samples taken before the emergence of asthma symptoms can discriminate the causes of the disease from the consequences. Recently, a genome-wide methylation study using cord blood mononuclear cells from neonates was performed to study development of childhood asthma by the age of 9 years [24]. The methylation level in the promoter region of the *SMAD3* gene was selectively associated with the development of asthma in children of asthmatic mothers. Furthermore, *SMAD3* promoter methylation in children of asthmatic mothers was significantly associated with neonatal IL1B production. These results suggest that epigenetic modification in response to the in utero environment promotes the developmental trajectory toward childhood asthma.

1.4 Conclusion

Candidate gene association studies of asthma have identified many risk alleles and loci. GWASs have further added a number of novel risk genes. Although the genetic basis for asthma is robust, each genomic variant identified by these strategies contributes only a small proportion to the heritability of asthma. This is partly due to the disease's heterogeneity, epistatic interactions, GxE interactions, and epigenetic modifications. Integrative applications of genome-wide epistatic and epigenetic approaches using an adequate number of samples with distinct asthma phenotypes are necessary for further elucidation of the causal variants behind the single-gene association studies. Genetic profiling for susceptibility to asthma and for the subsequent progression, severity, and therapeutic response of asthma is extremely useful for identifying individuals with asthma onset risk, modifying the disease progression, and developing personalized medicine.

Acknowledgments We would like to thank F. Miyamasu, associate professor of English for Medical Purposes, Medical English Communications Center, University of Tsukuba, for grammatical review and advice.

References

1. Polderman TJ, Benyamin B, de Leeuw CA, Sullivan PF, van Bochoven A, Visscher PM, et al. Meta-analysis of the heritability of human traits based on fifty years of twin studies. Nat Genet. 2015;47(7):702–9. https://doi.org/10.1038/ng.3285.
2. Pinero J, Bravo A, Queralt-Rosinach N, Gutierrez-Sacristan A, Deu-Pons J, Centeno E, et al. DisGeNET: a comprehensive platform integrating information on human disease-associated genes and variants. Nucleic Acids Res. 2017;45(D1):D833–900. https://doi.org/10.1093/nar/gkw943.
3. Vercelli D. Discovering susceptibility genes for asthma and allergy. Nat Rev Immunol. 2008;8(3):169–82. https://doi.org/10.1038/nri2257.
4. Kulkarni T, O'Reilly P, Antony VB, Gaggar A, Thannickal VJ. Matrix remodeling in pulmonary fibrosis and emphysema. Am J Respir Cell Mol Biol. 2016;54(6):751–60. https://doi.org/10.1165/rcmb.2015-0166PS.
5. Puxeddu I, Pang YY, Harvey A, Haitchi HM, Nicholas B, Yoshisue H, et al. The soluble form of a disintegrin and metalloprotease 33 promotes angiogenesis: implications for airway remodeling in asthma. J Allergy Clin Immunol. 2008;121(6):1400–6. https://doi.org/10.1016/j.jaci.2008.03.003.
6. Moffatt MF, Kabesch M, Liang L, Dixon AL, Strachan D, Heath S, et al. Genetic variants regulating ORMDL3 expression contribute to the risk of childhood asthma. Nature. 2007;448(7152):470–3. https://doi.org/10.1038/nature06014.
7. Andiappan AK, Sio YY, Lee B, Suri BK, Matta SA, Lum J, et al. Functional variants of 17q12-21 are associated with allergic asthma but not allergic rhinitis. J Allergy Clin Immunol. 2016;137(3):758–66.e3. https://doi.org/10.1016/j.jaci.2015.08.038.
8. Chen J, Miller M, Unno H, Rosenthal P, Sanderson MJ, Broide DH. Orosomucoid-like 3 (ORMDL3) upregulates airway smooth muscle proliferation, contraction, and Ca2+ oscillations in asthma. J Allergy Clin Immunol. 2017;142(1):207–218.e6. https://doi.org/10.1016/j.jaci.2017.08.015.
9. Das S, Miller M, Beppu AK, Mueller J, McGeough MD, Vuong C, et al. GSDMB induces an asthma phenotype characterized by increased airway responsiveness and remodeling without lung inflammation. Proc Natl Acad Sci U S A. 2016;113(46):13132–7. https://doi.org/10.1073/pnas.1610433113.
10. Pickrell JK, Berisa T, Liu JZ, Segurel L, Tung JY, Hinds DA. Detection and interpretation of shared genetic influences on 42 human traits. Nat Genet. 2016;48(7):709–17. https://doi.org/10.1038/ng.3570.

11. Ojiaku CA, Cao G, Zhu W, Yoo EJ, Shumyatcher M, Himes BE, et al. TGF-beta1 evokes human airway smooth muscle cell shortening and hyperresponsiveness via smad3. Am J Respir Cell Mol Biol. 2017;58(5):575–84. https://doi.org/10.1165/rcmb.2017-0247OC.
12. Kaneko Y, Masuko H, Sakamoto T, Iijima H, Naito T, Yatagai Y, et al. Asthma phenotypes in Japanese adults - their associations with the CCL5 and ADRB2 genotypes. Allergol Int. 2013;62(1):113–21. https://doi.org/10.2332/allergolint.12-OA-0467.
13. Yatagai Y, Hirota T, Sakamoto T, Yamada H, Masuko H, Kaneko Y, et al. Variants near the HLA complex group 22 gene (HCG22) confer increased susceptibility to late-onset asthma in Japanese populations. J Allergy Clin Immunol. 2016;138(1):281–3. https://doi.org/10.1016/j.jaci.2015.11.023.
14. Yatagai Y, Sakamoto T, Yamada H, Masuko H, Kaneko Y, Iijima H, et al. Genomewide association study identifies HAS2 as a novel susceptibility gene for adult asthma in a Japanese population. Clin Exp Allergy. 2014;44(11):1327–34. https://doi.org/10.1111/cea.12415.
15. Kabesch M, Schedel M, Carr D, Woitsch B, Fritzsch C, Weiland SK, et al. IL-4/IL-13 pathway genetics strongly influence serum IgE levels and childhood asthma. J Allergy Clin Immunol. 2006;117(2):269–74. https://doi.org/10.1016/j.jaci.2005.10.024.
16. Barnes KC, Grant A, Gao P, Baltadjieva D, Berg T, Chi P, et al. Polymorphisms in the novel gene acyloxyacyl hydroxylase (AOAH) are associated with asthma and associated phenotypes. J Allergy Clin Immunol. 2006;118(1):70–7. https://doi.org/10.1016/j.jaci.2006.03.036.
17. Millstein J, Conti DV, Gilliland FD, Gauderman WJ. A testing framework for identifying susceptibility genes in the presence of epistasis. Am J Hum Genet. 2006;78(1):15–27. https://doi.org/10.1086/498850.
18. Hizawa N, Maeda Y, Konno S, Fukui Y, Takahashi D, Nishimura M. Genetic polymorphisms at FCER1B and PAI-1 and asthma susceptibility. Clin Exp Allergy. 2006;36(7):872–6. https://doi.org/10.1111/j.1365-2222.2006.02413.x.
19. Murk W, DeWan AT. Genome-wide search identifies a gene-gene interaction between 20p13 and 2q14 in asthma. BMC Genet. 2016;17(1):102. https://doi.org/10.1186/s12863-016-0376-3.
20. Furler RL, Uittenbogaart CH. GLI2 regulates TGF-beta1 in human CD4+ T cells: implications in cancer and HIV pathogenesis. PLoS One. 2012;7(7):e40874. https://doi.org/10.1371/journal.pone.0040874.
21. Zambelli-Weiner A, Ehrlich E, Stockton ML, Grant AV, Zhang S, Levett PN, et al. Evaluation of the CD14/-260 polymorphism and house dust endotoxin exposure in the Barbados Asthma Genetics Study. J Allergy Clin Immunol. 2005;115(6):1203–9. https://doi.org/10.1016/j.jaci.2005.03.001.
22. Islam T, McConnell R, Gauderman WJ, Avol E, Peters JM, Gilliland FD. Ozone, oxidant defense genes, and risk of asthma during adolescence. Am J Respir Crit Care Med. 2008;177(4):388–95. https://doi.org/10.1164/rccm.200706-863OC.
23. Yang IV, Pedersen BS, Liu A, O'Connor GT, Teach SJ, Kattan M, et al. DNA methylation and childhood asthma in the inner city. J Allergy Clin Immunol. 2015;136(1):69–80. https://doi.org/10.1016/j.jaci.2015.01.025.
24. DeVries A, Wlasiuk G, Miller SJ, Bosco A, Stern DA, Lohman IC, et al. Epigenome-wide analysis links SMAD3 methylation at birth to asthma in children of asthmatic mothers. J Allergy Clin Immunol. 2017;140(2):534–42. https://doi.org/10.1016/j.jaci.2016.10.041.

Chapter 2
Group 2 Innate Lymphoid Cells and Asthma

Koichiro Asano

Abstract Group 2 innate lymphoid cells (ILC2s) do not express antigen-specific receptors or lineage-specific surface markers but produce large amounts of Th2 cytokines in response to interleukin (IL)-25 and IL-33 secreted from bronchial epithelial cells stimulated with protease-based allergens or infection with microorganisms. The number of ILC2s are increased and activated in the peripheral blood and airways of patients with asthma, especially with severe and/or eosinophilic forms. Corticosteroids can induce ILC2 apoptosis; however, these cells acquire corticosteroid resistance through activation of the Janus kinase/signal transducer and activator of transcription 5 pathway by thymic stromal lymphopoietin or IL-7. ILC2 activities are negatively regulated by interferons; however, lack of type I and III interferon synthesis in asthmatic airways exacerbates inflammation during respiratory viral infection.

Keywords Interleukin-33 · Thymic stromal lymphopoietin · Corticosteroids · Viral infection · Interferon

2.1 Introduction

2.1.1 Two Distinct Type-2 Immune Responses

Type 2 immune responses mediated by Th2 cytokines such as interleukin (IL)-4, IL-5, IL-13, and related molecules such as immunoglobulin (Ig)E elicit asthma-like pathologies in the airways, including eosinophilic inflammation, mucus hyperproduction, and

K. Asano (✉)
Division of Pulmonary Medicine, Department of Medicine, Tokai University School of Medicine, Kanagawa, Japan
e-mail: ko-asano@tokai-u.jp

A. Yokoyama (ed.), *Advances in Asthma*, Respiratory Disease Series: Diagnostic Tools and Disease Managements, https://doi.org/10.1007/978-981-13-2790-2_2

airway hyperresponsiveness. These responses can be induced in mice by repeated administration of antigens in conjunction with adjuvants such as alum; antigens are presented by dendritic cells to naïve T cells, inducing Th2 cell differentiation, Th2 cytokine production, and IgE class switching in B cells/plasma cells. These classic type-2 immune responses or "acquired-type allergies" require 2–3 weeks to develop in animal models.

Meanwhile, cytokines such as IL-25 and IL-33, produced by airway epithelial cells in response to allergens with protease activity, as well as viruses, fungi, and parasites, cause a similar asthma-like pathology with Th2 cytokine production in just a few days. This newly identified type 2 immune response occurs in the absence of allergens, T cells, or B cells and is termed "innate-type allergy" [1].

2.1.2 Group 2 Innate Lymphoid Cells (ILC2s)

Th2 cells are the predominant source of Th2 cytokines in acquired-type allergy, whereas group 2 innate lymphoid cells (ILC2), such as natural helper cells, play a major role in innate-type allergy. ILC2s are a subset of innate lymphoid cells that produce Th1, Th2, and Th17 cytokines and express receptors for IL-2 and IL-7 but, unlike T and B cells, do not express antigen-specific receptors or lineage-specific surface markers such as CD3, CD4, and CD19. Innate lymphoid cells are classified into three groups based on their phenotypical and functional characteristics: ILC1 (producing interferon (IFN)-γ), ILC2 (producing IL-5 and IL-13), and ILC3 (producing IL-17 and/or IL-22). They depend on specific transcription factors (T-box 21, GATA-binding protein 3, and RAR-related orphan receptor γt, respectively), for their development and function.

ILC2s are related to various physiological functions, from host defense against parasites to metabolic regulation in adipose tissue, and pathological conditions such as asthma, nasal polyps, and eczema. In the airways, ILC2s are activated in response to epithelial cell-derived cytokines such as IL-25, IL-33, and thymic stromal lymphopoietin (TSLP) and exhibit various biological functions ranging from the immunological modulation of eosinophils, T cells, and macrophages to airway remodeling and tissue repair (Fig. 2.1).

2.2 ILC2s in Patients with Asthma (Table 2.1)

2.2.1 ILC2s Are Increased in the Peripheral Blood and Airways of Patients with Asthma

The relationship between ILC2s and human asthma was first demonstrated in a small study in 2014 [2]. The proportion of ILC2s in peripheral blood mononuclear cells, examined in six patients with atopic asthma, was twice as high as that in healthy subjects or patients with allergic rhinitis. These results were consistent with studies showing that the proportion of ILC2s in the lymphocyte fraction of the peripheral blood was larger in patients with asthma than in healthy subjects [3, 4].

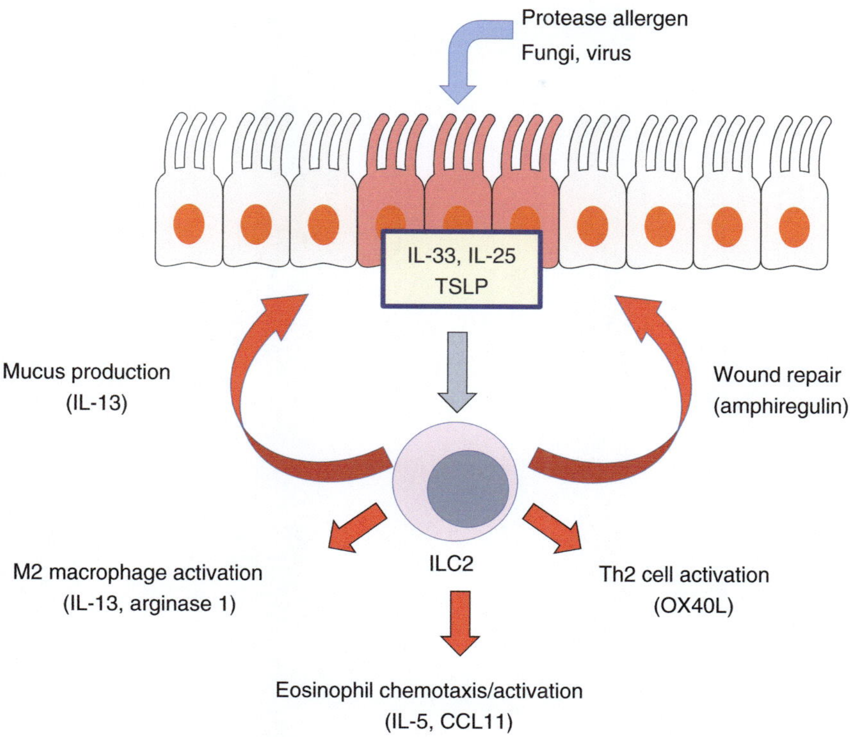

Fig. 2.1 Role of ILC2s in asthmatic airways. Bronchial epithelial cells express and release IL-25, IL-33, and TSLP in response to protease allergens and viral/fungal infections. These epithelial cell-derived cytokines activate ILC2s to proliferate and release cytokines/chemokines and growth factors such as IL-5, IL-13, C-C motif chemokine ligand 11 (CCL11), and amphiregulin, inducing airway inflammation and repair/remodeling

However, a pediatric study did not detect any difference in the proportion of peripheral blood ILC2s between children with severe asthma and subjects with respiratory tract infection [5]. Even in these children, however, the number of ILC2 cells in the sputum was greater in those with asthma. Another study investigated ILC2s in the lungs using bronchoalveolar lavage fluid (BALF) and found that the ILC2 cell ratio in the airways was increased in patients with asthma compared to subjects with non-asthmatic respiratory diseases, including chronic cough, bronchiectasis, mycobacterial infection, and chronic obstructive pulmonary disease [6].

2.2.2 *Increased ILC2 Numbers and Activation in More Severe Forms of Asthma*

The number of ILC2s in the peripheral blood and airways increases with increased asthma severity. The number of ILC2s in the peripheral blood and sputum was higher in patients with severe asthma than in patients with mild to moderate asthma

Table 2.1 Number of ILC2s in asthmatic patients

Studied subjects				ILC2 marker	Intracellular cytokine	Number of ILC2s			Ref.
Asthmatics	*n*	Controls	*n*			Blood	BALF	Sputum	
Atopic asthma	6	Healthy control	6	Lin$^-$CD127$^+$CRTH2$^+$		Increased			[2]
		Allergic rhinitis	6			Increased			
Asthma	52	Healthy control	34	Lin$^-$CD45^{hi}CD127$^+$CRTH2$^+$		Increased			[3]
Uncontrolled asthma	26	Healthy control	34		IL-5$^+$	NS			
					IL-13$^+$	Increased			
		Controlled asthma	26		IL-5$^+$	NS			
					IL-13$^+$	Increased			
Eosinophilic asthma	62	Healthy control	42	Lin$^-$CD127$^+$CRTH2$^+$		Increased			[4]
		Non-eosinophilic asthma	64			Increased			
Non-eosinophilic asthma	64	Healthy control	42			NS			
Severe pediatric asthma	11	Lower respiratory tract infection	16	Lin$^-$CD45$^+$CD127$^+$CRTH2$^+$		NS	increased		[5]
	13		6					Increased	
Asthma	38	Disease control	18	Lin$^-$FcεRI$^-$CD127$^+$ST2$^+$			increased		[6]
					IL-13$^+$		increased		
Severe asthma	25	Mild asthma	19	Lin$^-$FcεRI$^-$CD45$^+$CD127$^+$ST2$^+$		Increased		Increased	[7]
	25		9		IL-5$^+$	Increased			
					IL-13$^+$	Increased			
					IL-5$^+$IL-13$^+$	Increased			
	15		9		IL-5$^+$			Increased	
					IL-13$^+$			NS	
					IL-5$^+$IL-13$^+$			NS	

NS not significantly different, *BALF* bronchoalveolar lavage fluid, *CD127* IL-7 receptor α, *ST2* IL-33 receptor α

[7]. Another study found that the number of activated ILC2 cells expressing intracellular IL-13 was increased in poorly controlled asthma compared to stable disease [3]. In patients with uncontrolled asthma, 3 months of therapeutic intervention, including systemic corticosteroids, decreased the number of activated ILC2s to the levels observed in healthy individuals [3].

A remaining question is whether Th2 cells or ILC2s are the dominant source of Th2 cytokines, such as IL-5 and IL-13, in the airways or peripheral blood of patients with asthma. The proportion of IL-5/IL-13-positive cells is greater for ILC2s (up to 100%) than for $CD4^+$ T cells (less than 5%) [7]. Furthermore, the proportion of activated ILC2s increases with asthma severity while causing no changes in the number of IL-5/IL-13-positive $CD4^+$ T cells. However, the total number of $CD4^+$ T cells greatly exceeds that of ILC2s, and therefore, IL-5/IL-13-positive $CD4^+$ T cells in the sputum exceed the number of ILC2s even in patients with severe asthma.

2.2.3 ILC2s Are Increased in Eosinophilic Asthma

The asthma phenotype can also determine the degree of ILC2 involvement in its pathophysiology. The number of ILC2s in the sputum increases in asthma of eosinophilic phenotype. Patients with 3% sputum eosinophils or more display higher ILC2 ratios in their peripheral blood lymphocyte fractions than patients with non-eosinophilic asthma or healthy subjects [4]. Another study demonstrated that the number of activated ILC2s co-expressing IL-5 and IL-13 was more abundant in the sputum of patients with eosinophilic asthma than in those with non-eosinophilic asthma [7].

The association of ILC2s with eosinophilic asthma depends on the IL-33/IL-33 receptor axis. The IL-33 concentration is increased in the BALF of patients with asthma and is inversely correlated with pulmonary function [6]. Transcriptome analysis of sputum cells showed that the expression of interleukin 1 receptor like 1 (IL1RL1), the α-chain of the IL-33 receptor, is enhanced in patients with severe asthma with sputum eosinophils $\geq$1.49%, but not in patients with neutrophilic or paucigranulocytic forms [8]. IL1RL1 expression correlates well with the expression of IL-13-inducible Th2 gene signatures [8].

2.3 Corticosteroid Sensitivity of ILC2s

2.3.1 Corticosteroid Sensitivity of Murine and Human ILC2s

As discussed above, the number and activity of ILC2s in the peripheral blood and airways are increased in patients with severe asthma that cannot be controlled with standard inhaled corticosteroid treatment. This suggests that ILC2s are related to corticosteroid resistance in severe asthma. Kabata et al. investigated the corticosteroid sensitivity of mouse ILC2s isolated from the mesenteric fat-associated lymphoid cluster and the lungs by treating IL-33-stimulated ILC2s with dexamethasone. Corticosteroids induced ILC2 apoptosis and suppressed their cytokine production, suggesting that ILC2s are corticosteroid-sensitive Th2 cells [9]. The corticosteroid sensitivity of ILC2s in vivo was also confirmed using animal models of IL-33-dependent airway inflammation, in which IL-33 or a fungal extract (*Alternaria sp.*) was administered into the airways of mice [9, 10].

Liu and colleagues recently confirmed that human peripheral blood ILC2s are also corticosteroid-sensitive [11]. In their study, rather than exposing isolated ILC2s to dexamethasone, peripheral blood mononuclear cells were treated with dexamethasone for 5 days and then the ILC2 fraction was identified using flow cytometry. Treatment with dexamethasone reduced ILC2 viability from 64% to 45%, and the proportion of IL-5-positive cells among *Aspergillus* stimulated ILC2s from 84% to 9%. These in vitro and in vivo studies suggest that both human and murine ILC2s are susceptible to corticosteroids.

2.3.2 Murine and Human ILC2s Isolated from Asthmatic Airways Are Corticosteroid-Resistant

There is accumulating evidence that ILC2s in the airways of patients with asthma are relatively resistant to corticosteroids. This phenomenon was first demonstrated in mice [9]. Inhalation of an allergen (ovalbumin) by sensitized mice with coadministration of IL-33 led to eosinophilic inflammation, with activation of both Th2 cells and ILC2s in the airways. When corticosteroids were administered, Th2 cells immediately underwent apoptosis and were decreased significantly, but ILC2s remained activated, with Th2 cytokine production, causing sustained airway inflammation and bronchial hyperresponsiveness. Similarly, human ILC2s recovered from the BALF but not from the blood of patients with asthma are corticosteroid-resistant, with persistent IL-5 expression [11].

2.3.3 Mechanism of Corticosteroid Resistance Induction in Murine and Human ILC2s

To clarify the mechanism by which ILC2s acquire corticosteroid resistance in the airways of patients with asthma, Kabata et al. identified IL-2, IL-7, and TSLP as factors that inhibit the corticosteroid-dependent suppression of ILC2 proliferation and cytokine production [9]. Consistently, IL-7 and TSLP can induce corticosteroid resistance in human ILC2s [11]. TSLP is synthesized in the airways of mice and humans with asthma and may play a major role in inducing corticosteroid resistance in patients with severe asthma.

Both IL-7 and TSLP activate the Janus kinase (JAK)/signal transducer and activator of transcription (STAT) pathway via STAT5 phosphorylation by the IL-7 receptor-α chain, which displays enhanced expression in ILC2s treated with corticosteroids [11]. STAT5 inhibitors and the JAK inhibitor, tofacitinib, can suppress TSLP/IL-7-induced development of corticosteroid resistance in murine and human ILC2s [9, 11]. A screen of more than 1000 existing drugs identified an antipsychotic drug, pimozide, as a potent STAT5 inhibitor, which can reverse corticosteroid resistance in ILC2s treated with TSLP/IL-7 or recovered from BALF [9, 11]. Therefore, these drugs may serve as therapeutic agents for severe asthma.

2.4 Asthma Exacerbation due to Viral Infection and ILC2s

2.4.1 Airway IL-33/IL-25/TSLP Production During Viral Infection

Respiratory infection with rhinovirus, respiratory syncytial virus (RSV), and other viruses is the major cause of acute asthma exacerbation. When these viruses invade the airway epithelium, cytokines such as IL-25, IL-33, and TSLP are produced and released from epithelial cells [12]. To confirm whether similar phenomena occur in human airways, Jackson and colleagues experimentally infected volunteers with or without asthma with rhinovirus and collected nasal and bronchial epithelial lining fluid before and after infection to measure cytokine levels [13]. IL-33 concentrations in the nasal epithelial lining fluids increased after viral infection in both groups [13]. Interestingly, the concentrations of Th2 cytokines, such as IL-5 and IL-13, were elevated following viral infection only in volunteers with asthma, but not in healthy individuals [13].

Although airway epithelial cells are considered the main source of IL-33, other cell types may be involved in physiological and pathological IL-33 synthesis in the lungs. Two studies identified alveolar type II epithelial cells as a constitutive source of IL-33 in the murine lungs [14, 15]. Clara cells (serous cells), macrophages, and dendritic cells may produce IL-33 in the lungs after infection with viruses such as Sendai virus and RSV [14, 16].

2.4.2 IL-33/IL-25/TSLP-Mediated Exacerbation of Airway Inflammation During Viral Infection

There are several lines of evidence that IL-33 produced in the airways during viral infection can exacerbate inflammation. Secreted IL-33 can activate various inflammatory cells such as mast cells, T cells, and most of all, ILC2s. Administration of an IL-33 receptor-blocking antibody or IL-33 gene deficiency suppressed Th2 cytokine production and eosinophilic airway inflammation in a murine model of RSV infection [17, 18]. During rhinovirus infection, an anti-IL-33 antibody suppressed both eosinophilic inflammation and the increase in ILC2s [19, 20]. Dexamethasone similarly suppressed eosinophilic inflammation, but the administration of anti-IL-33 antibody, not corticosteroids, decreased the viral load itself [20].

IL-25 and TSLP are also synthesized in the airways during viral infection, but the roles of these cytokines in this condition remain less studied. IL-33 knockout mice display decreased airway inflammation, ILC2 activation, and Th2 cytokine production during RSV infection, and similar effects were observed when TSLP activity was inhibited by TSLP receptor gene knockout or anti-TSLP antibodies [17]. Airway inflammation in a rhinovirus infection model was also suppressed in TSLP receptor knockout mice [21]. These findings suggest that both IL-33 and TSLP are required for ILC2 activation during viral infection. Synergistic actions between IL-33 and TSLP may be related to their activation of IFN regulatory factor 4 in ILC2s, which induces the production of IL-9 to further activate IL-9 receptor-positive ILC2s in an autocrine fashion [15].

2.4.3 IFN Response in Healthy and Asthmatic Airways During Viral Infection

During experimental rhinovirus infection, IL-33 concentrations in the airways increased in both healthy volunteers and patients with asthma, but the concentrations of Th2 cytokines such as IL-5 and IL-13 were elevated only with asthma [13]. These discordant responses to IL-33 may be explained by differences in ILC2 negative regulation. In addition to receptors for IL-2, IL-7, IL-25, IL-33, and TSLP, which are necessary for ILC2 survival and activation, these cells also express receptors for IFNs, IL-10, IL-12, and IL-27, with previously unknown functions [22]. Recent studies have clarified that type I and type III IFNs, as well as IL-27, which can all activate STAT1, suppress ILC2 proliferation and Th2 cytokine production [22, 23]. During respiratory viral infection, a large amount of IFN is released from respiratory epithelial cells and plasmacytoid dendritic cells, which effectively eliminates virus-infected cells. These IFNs also suppress ILC2 functions activated by IL-33 and TSLP released from virus-infected epithelial cells (Fig. 2.2). In the absence of this negative regulatory system, influenza virus infection causes enhanced and prolonged airway inflammation in IFN receptor deficient mice [23]. In contrast, blocking IL-33 signaling during rhinovirus infection can enhance IFN production from airway epithelial cells and reduce the viral load [20]. In patients with asthma, however, this negative regulatory system is impaired due to reduced IFN synthesis in airway epithelial cells and plasmacytoid dendritic cells [24–27]. The restoration of IFN responses through IFN-β inhalation or IgE blockade has been shown to reduce the viral load and the exacerbation of asthma [28, 29].

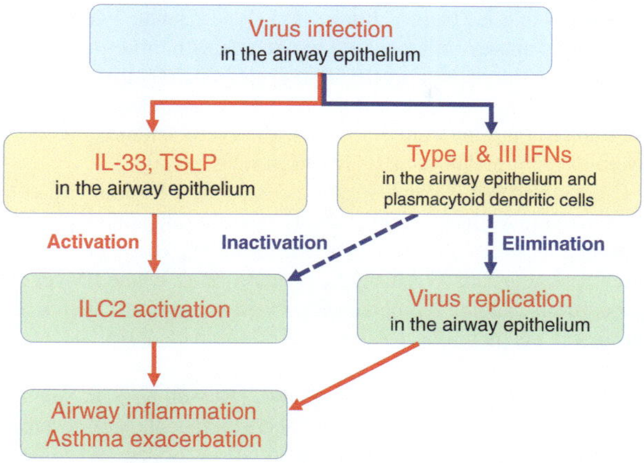

Fig. 2.2 Regulation of ILC2 activity during respiratory virus infection. Bronchial epithelial cells infected with rhinovirus or RSV synthesize IL-33 and TSLP, which activate ILC2s and induce airway inflammation. Bronchial epithelial and plasmacytoid dendritic cells synthesize type I and III IFNs during viral infection, which eliminate virus-infected epithelial cells and suppress ILC2s. In asthmatic airways, however, IFN production is impaired, and therefore, virus replication and ILC2 activation cannot be suppressed, causing exacerbated and prolonged airway inflammation

2.5 Conclusion

The discovery of ILC2s in 2010 significantly changed our understanding of asthma pathophysiology, which was previously limited to IgE-dependent allergic airway inflammation in atopic asthma. Today, we know how protease-based antigens, fungi, and viruses cause eosinophilic airway inflammation, how airway inflammation in severe asthma becomes corticosteroid-resistant, and how viral infection exacerbates eosinophilic airway inflammation in patients with asthma. Research on ILC2s is still rapidly progressing, hopefully enabling complete understanding of the role of ILC2s in asthma pathophysiology in the near future.

Acknowledgments This research was supported by the Japan Agency for Medical Research and Development (AMED) under grant number JP18ek0410026.

References

1. Yoshimoto T, Matsushita K. Innate-type and acquired-type allergy regulated by IL-33. Allergol Int. 2014;63(Suppl 1):3–11. https://doi.org/10.2332/allergolint.13-RA-0657.
2. Bartemes KR, Kephart GM, Fox SJ, Kita H. Enhanced innate type 2 immune response in peripheral blood from patients with asthma. J Allergy Clin Immunol. 2014;134:671–8.e4. https://doi.org/10.1016/j.jaci.2014.06.024.
3. Jia Y, Fang X, Zhu X, Bai C, Zhu L, Jin M, et al. IL-13+ type 2 innate lymphoid cells correlate with asthma control status and treatment response. Am J Respir Cell Mol Biol. 2016;55:675–83. https://doi.org/10.1165/rcmb.2016-0099OC.

4. Liu T, Wu J, Zhao J, Wang J, Zhang Y, Liu L, et al. Type 2 innate lymphoid cells: a novel biomarker of eosinophilic airway inflammation in patients with mild to moderate asthma. Respir Med. 2015;109:1391–6. https://doi.org/10.1016/j.rmed.2015.09.016.
5. Nagakumar P, Denney L, Fleming L, Bush A, Lloyd CM, Saglani S. Type 2 innate lymphoid cells in induced sputum from children with severe asthma. J Allergy Clin Immunol. 2016;137:624.e6–6.e6. https://doi.org/10.1016/j.jaci.2015.06.038.
6. Christianson CA, Goplen NP, Zafar I, Irvin C, Good JT Jr, Rollins DR, et al. Persistence of asthma requires multiple feedback circuits involving type 2 innate lymphoid cells and IL-33. J Allergy Clin Immunol. 2015;136:59–68.e14. https://doi.org/10.1016/j.jaci.2014.11.037.
7. Smith SG, Chen R, Kjarsgaard M, Huang C, Oliveria JP, O'Byrne PM, et al. Increased numbers of activated group 2 innate lymphoid cells in the airways of patients with severe asthma and persistent airway eosinophilia. J Allergy Clin Immunol. 2016;137:75–86.e8. https://doi.org/10.1016/j.jaci.2015.05.037.
8. Rossios C, Pavlidis S, Hoda U, Kuo CH, Wiegman C, Russell K, et al. Sputum transcriptomics reveal upregulation of IL-1 receptor family members in patients with severe asthma. J Allergy Clin Immunol. 2017;141(2):560–70. https://doi.org/10.1016/j.jaci.2017.02.045.
9. Kabata H, Moro K, Fukunaga K, Suzuki Y, Miyata J, Masaki K, et al. Thymic stromal lymphopoietin induces corticosteroid resistance in natural helper cells during airway inflammation. Nat Commun. 2013;4:2675. https://doi.org/10.1038/ncomms3675.
10. Walford HH, Lund SJ, Baum RE, White AA, Bergeron CM, Husseman J, et al. Increased ILC2s in the eosinophilic nasal polyp endotype are associated with corticosteroid responsiveness. Clin Immunol. 2014;155:126–35. https://doi.org/10.1016/j.clim.2014.09.007.
11. Liu S, Verma M, Michalec L, Liu W, Sripada A, Rollins D, et al. Steroid resistance of airway type 2 innate lymphoid cells from patients with severe asthma: The role of thymic stromal lymphopoietin. J Allergy Clin Immunol. 2017;141(1):257–268.e6. https://doi.org/10.1016/j.jaci.2017.03.032.
12. Kumar RK, Foster PS, Rosenberg HF. Respiratory viral infection, epithelial cytokines, and innate lymphoid cells in asthma exacerbations. J Leukoc Biol. 2014;96:391–6. https://doi.org/10.1189/jlb.3RI0314-129R.
13. Jackson DJ, Makrinioti H, Rana BM, Shamji BW, Trujillo-Torralbo MB, Footitt J, et al. IL-33-dependent type 2 inflammation during rhinovirus-induced asthma exacerbations in vivo. Am J Respir Crit Care Med. 2014;190:1373–82. https://doi.org/10.1164/rccm.201406-1039OC.
14. Byers DE, Alexander-Brett J, Patel AC, Agapov E, Dang-Vu G, Jin X, et al. Long-term IL-33-producing epithelial progenitor cells in chronic obstructive lung disease. J Clin Invest. 2013;123:3967–82. https://doi.org/10.1172/JCI65570.
15. Mohapatra A, Van Dyken SJ, Schneider C, Nussbaum JC, Liang HE, Locksley RM. Group 2 innate lymphoid cells utilize the IRF4-IL-9 module to coordinate epithelial cell maintenance of lung homeostasis. Mucosal Immunol. 2016;9:275–86. https://doi.org/10.1038/mi.2015.59.
16. Qi F, Wang D, Liu J, Zeng S, Xu L, Hu H, et al. Respiratory macrophages and dendritic cells mediate respiratory syncytial virus-induced IL-33 production in TLR3- or TLR7-dependent manner. Int Immunopharmacol. 2015;29:408–15. https://doi.org/10.1016/j.intimp.2015.10.022.
17. Stier MT, Bloodworth MH, Toki S, Newcomb DC, Goleniewska K, Boyd KL, et al. Respiratory syncytial virus infection activates IL-13-producing group 2 innate lymphoid cells through thymic stromal lymphopoietin. J Allergy Clin Immunol. 2016;138:814–24.e11. https://doi.org/10.1016/j.jaci.2016.01.050.
18. Zeng S, Wu J, Liu J, Qi F, Liu B. IL-33 receptor (ST2) signalling is important for regulation of Th2-mediated airway inflammation in a murine model of acute respiratory syncytial virus infection. Scand J Immunol. 2015;81:494–501. https://doi.org/10.1111/sji.12284.
19. Han M, Hong JY, Jaipalli S, Rajput C, Lei J, Hinde JL, et al. IFN-gamma blocks development of an asthma phenotype in rhinovirus-infected baby mice by inhibiting type 2 innate lymphoid cells. Am J Respir Cell Mol Biol. 2017;56:242–51. https://doi.org/10.1165/rcmb.2016-0056OC.

20. Werder RB, Zhang V, Lynch JP, Snape N, Upham JW, Spann K, et al. Chronic IL-33 expression predisposes to virus-induced asthma exacerbations by increasing type 2 inflammation and dampening antiviral immunity. J Allergy Clin Immunol. 2017;141(5):1607–1619.e9. https://doi.org/10.1016/j.jaci.2017.07.051.
21. Han M, Rajput C, Hong JY, Lei J, Hinde JL, Wu Q, et al. The innate cytokines IL-25, IL-33, and TSLP cooperate in the induction of type 2 innate lymphoid cell expansion and mucous metaplasia in rhinovirus-infected immature mice. J Immunol. 2017;199:1308–18. https://doi.org/10.4049/jimmunol.1700216.
22. Moro K, Kabata H, Tanabe M, Koga S, Takeno N, Mochizuki M, et al. Interferon and IL-27 antagonize the function of group 2 innate lymphoid cells and type 2 innate immune responses. Nat Immunol. 2016;17:76–86. https://doi.org/10.1038/ni.3309.
23. Duerr CU, McCarthy CD, Mindt BC, Rubio M, Meli AP, Pothlichet J, et al. Type I interferon restricts type 2 immunopathology through the regulation of group 2 innate lymphoid cells. Nat Immunol. 2016;17:65–75. https://doi.org/10.1038/ni.3308.
24. Contoli M, Message SD, Laza-Stanca V, Edwards MR, Wark PA, Bartlett NW, Kebadze T, Mallia P, Stanciu LA, Parker HL, et al. Role of deficient type III interferon-lambda production in asthma exacerbations. Nat Med. 2006;12:1023–6.
25. Durrani SR, Montville DJ, Pratt AS, Sahu S, DeVries MK, Rajamanickam V, et al. Innate immune responses to rhinovirus are reduced by the high-affinity IgE receptor in allergic asthmatic children. J Allergy Clin Immunol. 2012;130:489–95. https://doi.org/10.1016/j.jaci.2012.05.023.
26. Tversky JR, Le TV, Bieneman AP, Chichester KL, Hamilton RG, Schroeder JT. Human blood dendritic cells from allergic subjects have impaired capacity to produce interferon-alpha via Toll-like receptor 9. Clin Exp Allergy. 2008;38:781–8. https://doi.org/10.1111/j.1365-2222.2008.02954.x.
27. Wark PA, Johnston SL, Bucchieri F, Powell R, Puddicombe S, Laza-Stanca V, Holgate ST, Davies DE. Asthmatic bronchial epithelial cells have a deficient innate immune response to infection with rhinovirus. J Exp Med. 2005;201:937–47.
28. Teach SJ, Gill MA, Togias A, Sorkness CA, Arbes SJ Jr, Calatroni A, et al. Preseasonal treatment with either omalizumab or an inhaled corticosteroid boost to prevent fall asthma exacerbations. J Allergy Clin Immunol. 2015;136:1476–85. https://doi.org/10.1016/j.jaci.2015.09.008.
29. Djukanovic R, Harrison T, Johnston SL, Gabbay F, Wark P, Thomson NC, et al. The effect of inhaled IFN-beta on worsening of asthma symptoms caused by viral infections. A randomized trial. Am J Respir Crit Care Med. 2014;190:145–54. https://doi.org/10.1164/rccm.201312-2235OC.

Chapter 3
Cellular Mechanisms of Allergic Airway Inflammation

Koichi Takagi, Kentaro Machida, and Hiromasa Inoue

Abstract Asthma has long been considered to be driven by allergen-specific T helper 2 (Th2) responses. Although Th2 cytokines produced by Th2 cells play a central role in the induction and regulation of airway inflammation, clinical and basic studies have begun to shed light on the role of many types of cells. It is now well recognized that asthma is a multicellular disease, involving abnormal responses of many different cell types in the lung, including airway structural cells and innate and adaptive immune cells. A subpopulation of CD4+ T cells, such as Th1, Th17, and regulatory T cells (Tregs), has also been implicated in the regulation of airway inflammation. Airway epithelial cells and dendritic cells play an important role in promoting innate and adaptive immune responses in asthma. Group 2 innate lymphoid cells (ILC2s) stimulated by epithelial cell-derived cytokines, IL-25, IL-33, and thymic stromal lymphopoietin (TSLP), produce Th2 cytokines and have been reported to be involved in the induction of airway inflammation. Complementary experimental approaches including cultured cells, animal models, and human clinical studies have provided many insights into diverse cellular mechanisms in this complex disease.

Keywords Asthma · Airway inflammation · Airway structural cells · Innate and adaptive immune cells

K. Takagi · K. Machida · H. Inoue (✉)
Department of Pulmonary Medicine, Graduate School of Medical and Dental Sciences, Kagoshima University, Kagoshima, Japan
e-mail: inoue-pulm@umin.net

A. Yokoyama (ed.), *Advances in Asthma*, Respiratory Disease Series: Diagnostic Tools and Disease Managements, https://doi.org/10.1007/978-981-13-2790-2_3

3.1 Introduction

Asthma is a common heterogeneous disease with a chronic airway inflammation characterized by airway hyperresponsiveness (AHR), reversible airway obstruction and airway wall remodeling, and symptoms of recurrent wheezing, coughing, and shortness of breath. Airway inflammation due to asthma is associated with the infiltration of eosinophils, basophils, mast cells, and T helper (Th) cells into the airway submucosa. Airway epithelial cells are the first line of defense against inhaled environmental factors, such as pathogens and pollutants, and initiate airway inflammation, and these cells stimulated by inhaled allergens secrete the cytokines thymic stromal lymphopoietin (TSLP), interleukin-25 (IL-25), and IL-33, which act on subepithelial dendritic cells, mast cells, and innate lymphoid cells to recruit both innate and adaptive immune cells and initiate the release of type 2 cytokines IL-4, IL-5, IL-9, and IL-13.

These initial responses propagate to other cells such as T cells, B cells, and mast cells with the activation of airway structural cells such as airway smooth muscle cells, mucus goblet cells, and fibroblasts. Recently, group 2 innate lymphoid cells (ILC2s) have been recognized as important for the induction and regulation of allergic airway inflammation.

In this chapter, we will describe the cellular mechanisms of airway inflammation in asthma pathogenesis, mainly focusing on inflammatory cells and the cytokines produced by those cells. Here we review the recently published literature to discuss the potential pathological mechanisms regarding the onset and progressive severity of asthma with regard to disruption of the airway epithelial function.

3.2 Airway Structural Cells

Two types of airway cells, epithelial cells and smooth muscle cells, are considered to be crucial for asthma pathogenesis.

3.2.1 Airway Epithelial Cells

Airway epithelial cells lie at the interface between the host and the environment and form a barrier to the outside world; disruption of the barrier functions of the airway epithelium enhances the mucosal permeability of foreign substances in the airways. Epithelial cell activation is a key triggering event in the recognition of inhaled allergens that activates the local network of dendritic cells (DCs), which coordinate the subsequent immune response. The integrity of the epithelial barrier depends on apical tight junctions and adherens junctions that keep bronchial epithelial cells together and maintain their apicobasal polarity. Many studies have reported functional abnormalities of the airway epithelial cells in asthmatic patients, including

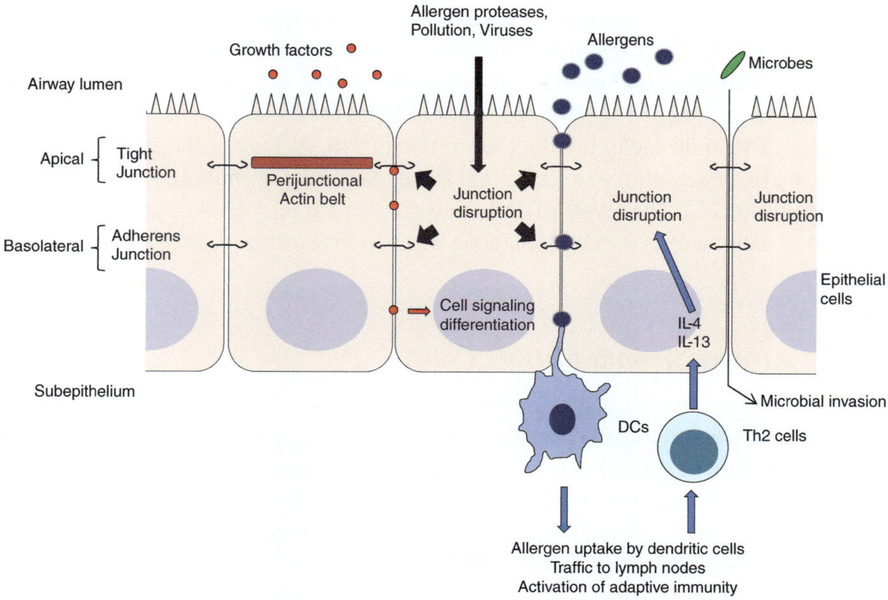

Fig. 3.1 Airway epithelial barrier function (*J Allergy Clin Immunol* 2014; 134:509–520, partial modification). Inhaled allergens, air pollutants, and respiratory viruses can cause dysfunction of the epithelial junction, resulting in enhanced mucosal permeability. This will result in a greater presentation of inhaled allergens and particles into the subepithelial space, facilitating innate and adaptive immune responses

the loss of tight junction proteins, a reduction in adherens junction proteins, and a reduction in desmosome length [1–3]. Increased barrier permeability might not only promote damage but also reduce the threshold for epithelial damage and the activation of a type 2 response (Fig. 3.1).

Recent studies have emphasized the importance of epithelial-derived cytokines that promote type 2 immune responses [4, 5]. Injured and activated airway epithelial cells release TSLP, IL-25, and IL-33, which act on DCs, mast cells, basophils, and ILC2s. Several reports have demonstrated that the levels of epithelium-derived cytokines are increased in asthmatic patients [6, 7]. IL-33, a member of the IL-1 cytokine family, has gained prominence in type 2 immunity since a recent genome-wide association study (GWAS) showed the genetic association of both IL-33 and its receptor, ST2 (IL-1 receptor-like 1), with asthma development [5, 8]. The levels of IL-33 in bronchoalveolar lavage fluid (BALF) were increased in asthmatic subjects and negatively correlated with lung function [9]. IL-25 belongs to the IL-17 cytokine family and is secreted by Th2 cells, mast cells, basophils, and eosinophils, as well as epithelial cells. The expression of IL-25 has been reported to be increased in the epithelial cells of patients with Th2-high asthma [10]. IL-33 activates lung ILC2s to produce large quantities of IL-5 and IL-13 in vitro. IL-25 and TSLP synergistically enhance cytokine production by ILC2s [11]. IL-25 and IL-33 also promote the expansion and/or migration of lung ILC2s [12, 13]. IL-33 is probably more potent than IL-25 for inducing ILC2 cell expansion [14]. In mice, epithelium-derived cytokines, such as IL-33 and IL-25, induce eosinophilic airway inflammation independent of acquired immunity. TSLP, an IL-7-like cytokine, stimulates the DC maturation that facilitates the generation of effector T cells and triggers the release of Th2 cytokines. A variety of stimuli, including double-stranded RNA and allergens, increase TSLP expression in airway epithelial cells, and these reactions are enhanced by inflammatory cytokines [15]. The levels of TSLP expression are increased in the airway epithelium of asthmatics, especially in those with severe asthma.

3.2.2 Airway Smooth Muscle Cells

The bands of smooth muscle present in both central and peripheral airways and the contraction of these smooth muscles, which can be induced by the release of acetylcholine from efferent parasympathetic nerves or by the release of histamine and cysteinyl leukotrienes from mast cells and basophils, cause airway narrowing. AHR is a characteristic feature of asthma. Asthmatic patients have a marked increase in sensitivity to these contractile agonists that can readily be demonstrated by a dramatic increase in airway resistance and associated drops in maximal expiratory airflow rates during forced expiratory maneuvers [16]. Several studies have suggested that cytokines released from T cells can contribute to AHR in allergic asthma [17]. The Th2 cytokine IL-13 can induce AHR when administered into the airways of mice [18, 19], and chronic allergen challenge or direct administration of IL-13 into airways of mice increased RhoA expression, which is a critical effector of airway smooth muscle cell contraction [20]. Studies have demonstrated suppressor of cytokine signaling (SOCS) 1 and 3, negative regulators of cytokine signaling, as potentially important in enhancing allergic inflammation [21, 22]. A recent study suggested that IL-17 can also increase airway smooth muscle contractility and airway narrowing by the induction of RhoA in airway smooth muscle cells [23]. Repeated bronchoconstriction induced by either allergens or methacholine increased TGF-β immunoreactivity within the airway epithelium and increased the thickness of the subepithelial collagen layer to promote airway remodeling independent of airway inflammation [24].

3.3 Innate and Adaptive Immune Cells

3.3.1 Dendritic Cells (DCs) (Fig. 3.2)

DCs play critical roles in initiating and directing immune responses, serving as sentinels at the mucosal surfaces, where they constantly sample the antigens at the interface between the external and internal environment. DCs migrate to the draining lymph nodes and present antigen to naïve and memory T cells and play primary

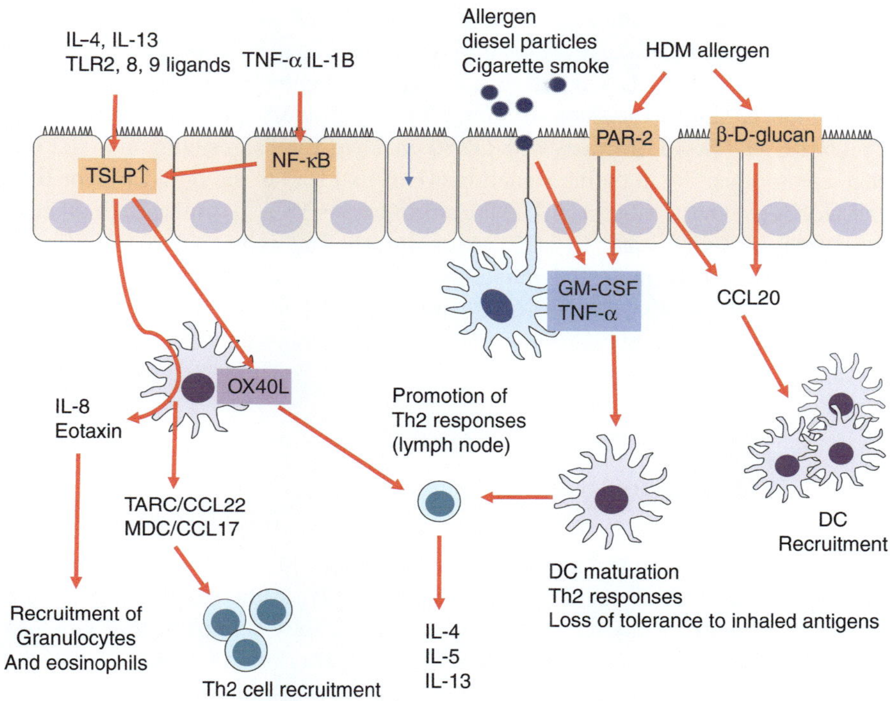

Fig. 3.2 Interaction between airway epithelial cells and DCs relevant to the pathogenesis of allergic asthma (*J Allergy Clin Immunol* 2012; 129:889–901, partial modification). The cross talk between epithelial cells and DCs through CCL2, CCL20, TSLP, OX40L, GM-CSF, and others promotes inflammatory cytokine production and the recruitment of inflammatory cells, skewing DCs toward a pro-Th2 phenotype

roles in determining the nature of T-lymphocyte differentiation in the face of allergen exposure [25]. DCs can drive the differentiation of naïve T cells into Th2 cells, which release Th2 cytokines, IL-4, IL-5, and IL-13, key mediators of induction allergic airway inflammation.

Significant increases in the numbers of airway DCs after exposure to allergens have been observed in both murine and rat models of asthma [26, 27]. It has been demonstrated that the placement of OVA-pulsed DCs directly into the airways of naïve animals results in not only OVA sensitization but also an ensuing Th2 response and AHR after rechallenge with OVA in the airways [28]. Conversely, the depletion of DCs from OVA-sensitized mice abrogates aeroallergen-induced AHR and that repletion of these cells restores the asthma phenotype in the animal models of allergic asthma [29]. All of these observations together support the critical roles of DCs in both the development and maintenance of allergen-induced airway inflammation and AHR in murine models.

C-C motif chemokine ligand 2 (CCL2), CCL20, TSLP, the OX40 ligand (OX40L), and the granulocyte-macrophage colony-stimulating factor (GM-CSF) produced by activated epithelial cells influence DC function. CCL2 and CCL20 attract monocytes and immature DCs to the lung. TSLP promotes allergic inflammation by inducing DCs to drive the differentiation of naïve CD4+ T cells into Th2 cells that secrete IL-4, IL-5, and IL-13. Th2 cell differentiation is mediated through TSLP-induced DC expression of the TNF superfamily protein OX40L [30]. DC-expressed OX40L interacts with OX40 on naïve T cells, resulting in a Th2 lineage commitment by initiating signaling events that lead to the production of IL-4 and GATA-3 transcription [31]. TSLP also stimulates DCs to synthesize high concentrations of CCL17 and CCL22, which attracts Th2 cells [30]. GM-CSF also stimulates DCs to promote Th2 immunity. Exposure to allergen-derived proteases induces airway epithelial cell GM-CSF secretion. GM-CSF induces DC maturation, resulting in the increased expression of DC costimulatory molecules and increased priming of T-lymphocyte responses.

3.3.2 CD4$^+$ T cells

It is now generally accepted that CD4$^+$ T cells are functionally divided into various subsets: Th1, Th2, Th17, and Tregs (regulatory T cells). Although plasticity among these subsets is frequently reported, these cells are mainly defined by the cytokines they produce together with their signature master transcription factors.

Typically, asthma is recognized as an inflammatory disorder of the airway associated with the Th2 cell-dependent promotion of IgE production and the recruitment of mast cells and eosinophils. However, accumulating evidence indicates that asthma is a more complicated heterogeneous disease, and a T cell subset other than Th2 cells, such as Th1, Th17, and Tregs, is involved in the development of airway inflammation in asthma.

3.3.2.1 Th2 Cells (Fig. 3.3)

Antigen-presenting cells, such as DCs and basophils, induce the differentiation of naïve CD4+ cells into Th2 cells by activating GATA3 through sirtuin-1, a class 3 histone deacetylase [32]. Allergen-specific Th2 cells are thought to be present in the lungs of almost all patients with asthma, particularly patients with allergic asthma [33]. In mouse models of allergic asthma, mice can be sensitized to a number of foreign proteins, such as ovalbumin (OVA), house dust mite (HDM) extract, and ragweed pollen, by immunization with adjuvants such as alum [34]. This immunization results in a Th2-polarized response and enhanced allergen-specific IgE production. Once sensitization has occurred, repeated administration of the allergen into the lungs leads to the common features of human allergic asthma, such as airway eosinophilia, mucus secretion, goblet cell hyperplasia, AHR, and airway remodeling. Th2 cells play an important role in the development and pathology of asthma. IL-4, IL-5, IL-9, and IL-13, produced by Th2 cells, are recognized as important cytokines for the induction of allergic airway inflammation in asthma. IL-4 is essential for the differentiation of Th2 cells and induces the secretion of IgE from B cells, the proliferation of mast cells,

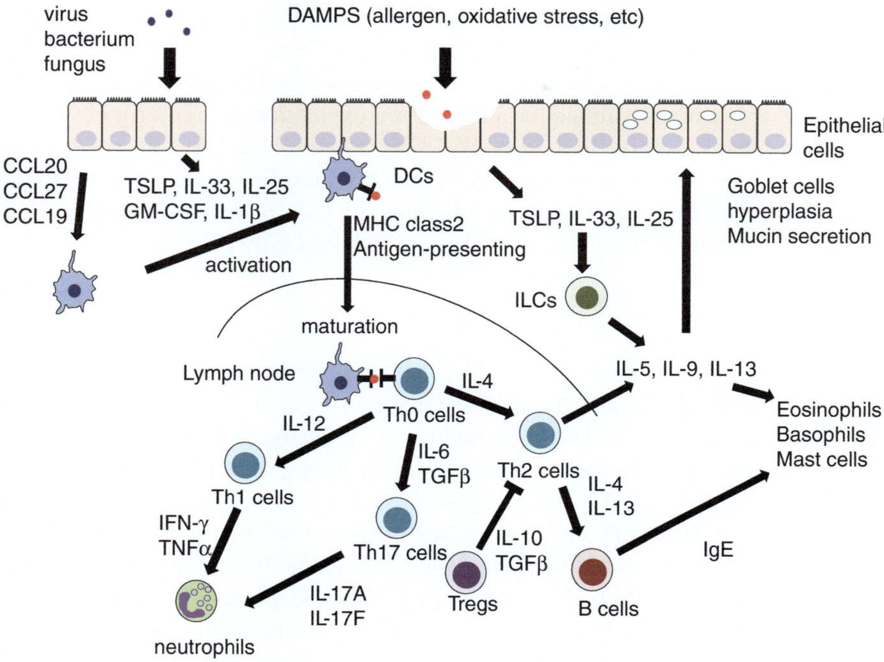

Fig. 3.3 Innate and adaptive immune responses in asthma. Epithelium-derived cytokines stimulate ILC2 and induce the production of type 2 cytokines. DCs migrate to regional lymph nodes to activate an allergen-specific CD4+ T-cell response

and eosinophil accumulation by the enhancement of vascular cell adhesion molecule-1 (VCAM-1) in vascular endothelial cells. IL-5 induces eosinophilic airway inflammation by facilitating the differentiation, maturity, and activation of eosinophils [35]. IL-5 is also thought to be associated with airway remodeling because it induces the deposition of extracellular matrix proteins under airway epithelial tissues through the production of TGF-beta from eosinophils. IL-9 induces mast cell differentiation, proliferation, activation, and accumulation in the airways and enhances goblet cell hyperplasia and mucus production. IL-13 induces epithelial eotaxin expression, eosinophil influx in the airways, goblet cell hyperplasia with mucus hypersecretion, and AHR. Glucocorticoid is reported not to be sufficient to suppress IL-13-induced responses, such as AHR [20]. These findings support the notion that Th2 cells and their cytokines play major roles not only in the induction of airway inflammation associated with asthma but also in steroid-resistant severe asthma.

3.3.2.2 Th1 Cells

Naïve $CD4^+$ cells were differentiated to Th1 cells in the presence of IL-12. Th1 cells were thought to inhibit allergic reactions by the Th1/Th2 paradigm, and IFN-γ produced by Th1 cells was indicated to inhibit the infiltration of eosinophils in the airway and AHR. On the other hand, a previous report demonstrated that the intratracheal administration of antigen-specific Th1 cells exacerbated eosinophilic airway inflammation in mice [36]. Other reports demonstrated that Th1 cells stimulated by an antigen in the presence of IL-18 produced IL-13 [37], and chronic repetitive excessive antigen stimulation induced the expression of transcription factor E4BP4 and gave the ability to produce IL-13 on Th1 cells [38]. Th1 cells are thought to play the roles of both induction and inhibition of allergic airway inflammation, depending on differences in the local inflammatory environment. The contribution of Th1 cells in the pathogenesis of asthma has not been fully elucidated.

3.3.2.3 Th17 Cells

Naïve $CD4^+$ cells differentiated to Th17 cells, which produce IL-17-A, IL-17-F, and IL-22 in the presence of TGF-β, IL-6, and IL-23, respectively. Th17 cells have been strongly linked with neutrophilic inflammation in autoimmune disease. Recently, it has been suggested that Th17 cells are involved in the pathogenesis of asthma and corticosteroid insensitivity, and this has led to the development of mouse models that overexpress IL-17. Several groups have reported that the number of Th17 cells and the expression of both IL-17A and IL-17F in the airway are high in severe asthma, in association with neutrophil infiltration, poor lung function, and steroid insensitivity [39, 40]. Although further investigation of the role of Th17 cells and their cytokines in airway inflammation in asthma is needed, Th17 cells are thought to be associated with severe asthma because they induce neutrophilic inflammation.

3.3.2.4 Regulatory T cells (Tregs)

Tregs were initially described as a small population of $CD4^+$ T cells expressing the IL-2 receptor α chain (CD25), and their capacity to regulate immune responses helps maintain homeostasis and self-tolerance. The $Foxp3^+$Treg can be divided into two distinct groups, naturally occurring Tregs (nTregs) derived from the thymus and secondary lymphoid-derived inducible Tregs (iTregs) that develop from peripheral naïve T cells, both expressing forkhead box P3 (Foxp3), as a specific Treg marker essential to their development and function [40, 41]. Functionally, Tregs exhibit a potent suppressive capacity to induce tolerance. Treg suppressive functions are mediated through several different mechanisms, including the release of immunoregulatory cytokines IL-10 and TGF-β and cell-to-cell contact via surface molecules such as CTLA-4 [42, 43]. Allergic diseases reflect a failure to develop tolerance of specific allergens. Murine models have provided strong evidence for an important role for Tregs in suppressing allergic airway inflammation.

In humans, it has been demonstrated that a reduced frequency of Tregs is associated with airway inflammation. The balance between Tregs and Th2 cells in the peripheral blood is different in healthy subjects as compared with atopic asthmatic patients [44]. Pediatric asthmatic patients were found to have a lower percentage of Tregs in the

BALF as compared with healthy children, and inhaled corticosteroid treatment increased the percentage of Tregs in pediatric asthmatic patients [45]. Tregs have been shown to be a suppressive regulator of airway inflammation to promote and maintain tolerance to allergens by regulating both innate and adaptive immune responses.

3.3.3 Group 2 Lymphoid Cell, Innate Lymphoid Cells (ILCs) (Fig. 3.3)

Recent discoveries have led to the identification of a novel group of immune cells, the innate lymphoid cells (ILCs). On the basis of their transcriptional requirements and the types of cytokines produced, ILCs can be divided into three major groups, ILC1, ILC2, and ILC3, that are similar to Th1, Th2, and Th17 cells, respectively [46].

ILC2s produce a large amount of type 2 cytokines, such as IL-5 and IL-13 [47], to respond to the stimulation of epithelial-derived cytokines, IL-25, IL-33 [13, 48], and TSLP [49]. Experimental models of type 2 immunity have led to a rapid increase in knowledge about ILC2s and indicate that they might play a role in the pathophysiology of asthma. Inhalation of IL-33 and IL-25 induces eosinophilic airway inflammation accompanied by AHR in mice, even recombination-activating gene (Rag)-/-mice, which lack T cells, B cells, and natural killer T cells [11, 50]. These findings show that ILC2s induce eosinophilic airway inflammation independent of acquired immunity upon activation by epithelium-derived cytokines. Recent studies showed that genetic polymorphisms in the gene encoding IL-33, which is a major activator of ILC2s, and its receptor ST2 are strongly linked to asthma development in GWASs [5]. It was shown that the expression of TSLP, IL-25, and IL-33 is increased in the airways of asthmatic patients [17, 18] and the number of total ILCs and type 2 cytokine-producing ILCs in peripheral blood and sputum were significantly increased in patients with systemic steroid-dependent severe eosinophilic asthma as compared with those with mild asthma [51]. ILC2s contribute not only to the initiation of innate allergic airway inflammation but also to the enhancement of allergic inflammation by interacting with other immune cells. For example, ILC2s have been reported to have a direct effect on Th2 cell activation through the OX40 ligand [52] and MHC class2 [53], expressing on ILC2s. Recent studies suggest that ILC2s also play important roles in steroid-resistant severe asthma [54]. These studies indicated that ILC2s play a pivotal role in the initiation and enhancement of allergic airway inflammation.

3.4 Conclusion

We reviewed cellular mechanisms associated with airway inflammation in asthma. Although the Th2 paradigm provides a reasonable foundation for understanding allergic diseases, including asthma, accumulated evidence demonstrates that asthma is a heterogeneous disease with multiple phenotypes representing a different pathophysiology involving many cell types. Disruption of the airway epithelial cell barrier function has been implicated in the induction of airway inflammation. Airway epithelial cells also play a pivotal role in activating both innate and adaptive immunity. DCs are present at the pulmonary mucosal interface, where they serve as innate sensors of foreign antigens and transmit this information to the immune system. Th2 cells play a central role in inducing airway inflammation in asthma, but another subset, Th1 and Th17, also plays several roles in the pathogenesis of asthma, especially the severe phenotype. Tregs have suppressive effects on immune response, and an imbalance in the frequency of Tregs and Th2 cells is implicated in airway inflammation. It has also been clarified that newly discovered ILC2 cells are implicated in the initiation and propagation of airway inflammation. It is expected that elucidating the cellular mechanisms involved in airway inflammation and further understanding the pathogenesis of asthma will lead to the development of novel therapeutic agents for the treatment of patients with severe asthma.

References

1. de Boer WI, Sharma HS, Baelemans SM, Hoogsteden HC, Lambrecht BN, Braunstahl GJ. Altered expression of epithelial junctional proteins in atopic asthma: possible role in inflammation. Can J Physiol Pharmacol. 2008;86(3):105–12. https://doi.org/10.1139/y08-004.
2. Shahana S, Bjornsson E, Ludviksdottir D, Janson C, Nettelbladt O, Venge P, et al. Ultrastructure of bronchial biopsies from patients with allergic and non-allergic asthma. Respir Med. 2005;99(4):429–43. https://doi.org/10.1016/j.rmed.2004.08.013.
3. Georas SN, Rezaee F. Epithelial barrier function: at the front line of asthma immunology and allergic airway inflammation. J Allergy Clin Immunol. 2014;134(3):509–20. https://doi.org/10.1016/j.jaci.2014.05.049.
4. Ziegler SF. Thymic stromal lymphopoietin and allergic disease. J Allergy Clin Immunol. 2012;130(4):845–52. https://doi.org/10.1016/j.jaci.2012.07.010.
5. Grotenboer NS, Ketelaar ME, Koppelman GH, Nawijn MC. Decoding asthma: translating genetic variation in IL33 and IL1RL1 into disease pathophysiology. J Allergy Clin Immunol. 2013;131(3):856–65. https://doi.org/10.1016/j.jaci.2012.11.028.
6. Prefontaine D, Nadigel J, Chouiali F, Audusseau S, Semlali A, Chakir J, et al. Increased IL-33 expression by epithelial cells in bronchial asthma. J Allergy Clin Immunol. 2010;125(3):752–4. https://doi.org/10.1016/j.jaci.2009.12.935.
7. Shikotra A, Choy DF, Ohri CM, Doran E, Butler C, Hargadon B, et al. Increased expression of immunoreactive thymic stromal lymphopoietin in patients with severe asthma. J Allergy Clin Immunol. 2012;129(1):104–11.e1. https://doi.org/10.1016/j.jaci.2011.08.031.
8. Tamari M, Tanaka S, Hirota T. Genome-wide association studies of allergic diseases. Allergol Int. 2013;62(1):21–8. https://doi.org/10.2332/allergolint.13-RAI-0539.
9. Christianson CA, Goplen NP, Zafar I, Irvin C, Good JT Jr, Rollins DR, et al. Persistence of asthma requires multiple feedback circuits involving type 2 innate lymphoid cells and IL-33. J Allergy Clin Immunol. 2015;136(1):59–68.e14. https://doi.org/10.1016/j.jaci.2014.11.037.
10. Sharma K. IL-18 attenuates experimental choroidal neovascularization as a potential therapy for wet age-related macular degeneration. Sci Transl Med 6, 230ra44 (2014). Ann Neurosci. 2014;21(4):150. https://doi.org/10.5214/ans.0972.7531.210407.
11. Halim TY, Krauss RH, Sun AC, Takei F. Lung natural helper cells are a critical source of Th2 cell-type cytokines in protease allergen-induced airway inflammation. Immunity. 2012;36(3):451–63. https://doi.org/10.1016/j.immuni.2011.12.020.

12. Barlow JL, Bellosi A, Hardman CS, Drynan LF, Wong SH, Cruickshank JP, et al. Innate IL-13-producing nuocytes arise during allergic lung inflammation and contribute to airways hyperreactivity. J Allergy Clin Immunol. 2012;129(1):191–8.e1. https://doi.org/10.1016/j.jaci.2011.09.041.
13. Price AE, Liang HE, Sullivan BM, Reinhardt RL, Eisley CJ, Erle DJ, et al. Systemically dispersed innate IL-13-expressing cells in type 2 immunity. Proc Natl Acad Sci U S A. 2010;107(25):11489–94. https://doi.org/10.1073/pnas.1003988107.
14. Barlow JL, Peel S, Fox J, Panova V, Hardman CS, Camelo A, et al. IL-33 is more potent than IL-25 in provoking IL-13-producing nuocytes (type 2 innate lymphoid cells) and airway contraction. J Allergy Clin Immunol. 2013;132(4):933–41. https://doi.org/10.1016/j.jaci.2013.05.012.
15. Hui CC, Murphy DM, Neighbour H, Al-Sayegh M, O'Byrne S, Thong B, et al. T cell-mediated induction of thymic stromal lymphopoietin in differentiated human primary bronchial epithelial cells. Clin Exp Allergy. 2014;44(7):953–64. https://doi.org/10.1111/cea.12330.
16. Boushey HA, Holtzman MJ, Sheller JR, Nadel JA. Bronchial hyperreactivity. Am Rev Respir Dis. 1980;121(2):389–413. https://doi.org/10.1164/arrd.1980.121.2.389.
17. Locksley RM. Asthma and allergic inflammation. Cell. 2010;140(6):777–83. https://doi.org/10.1016/j.cell.2010.03.004.
18. Grunig G, Warnock M, Wakil AE, Venkayya R, Brombacher F, Rennick DM, et al. Requirement for IL-13 independently of IL-4 in experimental asthma. Science. 1998;282(5397):2261–3.
19. Kibe A, Inoue H, Fukuyama S, Machida K, Matsumoto K, Koto H, et al. Differential regulation by glucocorticoid of interleukin-13-induced eosinophilia, hyperresponsiveness, and goblet cell hyperplasia in mouse airways. Am J Respir Crit Care Med. 2003;167(1):50–6. https://doi.org/10.1164/rccm.2110084.
20. Goto K, Chiba Y, Matsusue K, Hattori Y, Maitani Y, Sakai H, et al. The proximal STAT6 and NF-kappaB sites are responsible for IL-13- and TNF-alpha-induced RhoA transcriptions in human bronchial smooth muscle cells. Pharmacol Res. 2010;61(5):466–72. https://doi.org/10.1016/j.phrs.2009.12.001.
21. Seki Y, Inoue H, Nagata N, Hayashi K, Fukuyama S, Matsumoto K, et al. SOCS-3 regulates onset and maintenance of T(H)2-mediated allergic responses. Nat Med. 2003;9(8):1047–54. https://doi.org/10.1038/nm896.
22. Fukuyama S, Nakano T, Matsumoto T, Oliver BG, Burgess JK, Moriwaki A, et al. Pulmonary suppressor of cytokine signaling-1 induced by IL-13 regulates allergic asthma phenotype. Am J Respir Crit Care Med. 2009;179(11):992–8. https://doi.org/10.1164/rccm.200806-992OC.
23. Sahoo SK, Shaikh SA, Sopariwala DH, Bal NC, Periasamy M. Sarcolipin protein interaction with sarco(endo)plasmic reticulum Ca2+ ATPase (SERCA) is distinct from phospholamban protein, and only sarcolipin can promote uncoupling of the SERCA pump. J Biol Chem. 2013;288(10):6881–9. https://doi.org/10.1074/jbc.M112.436915.
24. Grainge CL, Lau LC, Ward JA, Dulay V, Lahiff G, Wilson S, et al. Effect of bronchoconstriction on airway remodeling in asthma. N Engl J Med. 2011;364(21):2006–15. https://doi.org/10.1056/NEJMoa1014350.
25. Bates EE, Dieu MC, Ravel O, Zurawski SM, Patel S, Bridon JM, et al. CD40L activation of dendritic cells down-regulates DORA, a novel member of the immunoglobulin superfamily. Mol Immunol. 1998;35(9):513–24.
26. Hammad H, Chieppa M, Perros F, Willart MA, Germain RN, Lambrecht BN. House dust mite allergen induces asthma via Toll-like receptor 4 triggering of airway structural cells. Nat Med. 2009;15(4):410–6. https://doi.org/10.1038/nm.1946.
27. van Rijt LS, Prins JB, Leenen PJ, Thielemans K, de Vries VC, Hoogsteden HC, et al. Allergen-induced accumulation of airway dendritic cells is supported by an increase in CD31(hi) Ly-6C(neg) bone marrow precursors in a mouse model of asthma. Blood. 2002;100(10):3663–71. https://doi.org/10.1182/blood-2002-03-0673.
28. Sung S, Rose CE, Fu SM. Intratracheal priming with ovalbumin- and ovalbumin 323-339 peptide-pulsed dendritic cells induces airway hyperresponsiveness, lung eosinophilia, goblet cell hyperplasia, and inflammation. J Immunol. 2001;166(2):1261–71.

29. van Rijt LS, Jung S, Kleinjan A, Vos N, Willart M, Duez C, et al. In vivo depletion of lung CD11c+ dendritic cells during allergen challenge abrogates the characteristic features of asthma. J Exp Med. 2005;201(6):981–91. https://doi.org/10.1084/jem.20042311.
30. Ito T, Wang YH, Duramad O, Hori T, Delespesse GJ, Watanabe N, et al. TSLP-activated dendritic cells induce an inflammatory T helper type 2 cell response through OX40 ligand. J Exp Med. 2005;202(9):1213–23. https://doi.org/10.1084/jem.20051135.
31. So T, Song J, Sugie K, Altman A, Croft M. Signals from OX40 regulate nuclear factor of activated T cells c1 and T cell helper 2 lineage commitment. Proc Natl Acad Sci U S A. 2006;103(10):3740–5. https://doi.org/10.1073/pnas.0600205103.
32. Colley T, Mercado N, Kunori Y, Brightling C, Bhavsar PK, Barnes PJ, et al. Defective sirtuin-1 increases IL-4 expression through acetylation of GATA-3 in patients with severe asthma. J Allergy Clin Immunol. 2016;137(5):1595–7.e7. https://doi.org/10.1016/j.jaci.2015.10.013.
33. Robinson DS, Hamid Q, Ying S, Tsicopoulos A, Barkans J, Bentley AM, et al. Predominant TH2-like bronchoalveolar T-lymphocyte population in atopic asthma. N Engl J Med. 1992;326(5):298–304. https://doi.org/10.1056/nejm199201303260504.
34. Kim HY, DeKruyff RH, Umetsu DT. The many paths to asthma: phenotype shaped by innate and adaptive immunity. Nat Immunol. 2010;11(7):577–84. https://doi.org/10.1038/ni.1892.
35. Fulkerson PC, Rothenberg ME. Targeting eosinophils in allergy, inflammation and beyond. Nat Rev Drug Discov. 2013;12(2):117–29. https://doi.org/10.1038/nrd3838.
36. Randolph DA, Stephens R, Carruthers CJ, Chaplin DD. Cooperation between Th1 and Th2 cells in a murine model of eosinophilic airway inflammation. J Clin Invest. 1999;104(8):1021–9. https://doi.org/10.1172/jci7631.
37. Hayashi N, Yoshimoto T, Izuhara K, Matsui K, Tanaka T, Nakanishi K. T helper 1 cells stimulated with ovalbumin and IL-18 induce airway hyperresponsiveness and lung fibrosis by IFN-gamma and IL-13 production. Proc Natl Acad Sci U S A. 2007;104(37):14765–70. https://doi.org/10.1073/pnas.0706378104.
38. Motomura Y, Kitamura H, Hijikata A, Matsunaga Y, Matsumoto K, Inoue H, et al. The transcription factor E4BP4 regulates the production of IL-10 and IL-13 in CD4+ T cells. Nat Immunol. 2011;12(5):450–9. https://doi.org/10.1038/ni.2020.
39. Kudo M, Melton AC, Chen C, Engler MB, Huang KE, Ren X, et al. IL-17A produced by alphabeta T cells drives airway hyper-responsiveness in mice and enhances mouse and human airway smooth muscle contraction. Nat Med. 2012;18(4):547–54. https://doi.org/10.1038/nm.2684.
40. Barczyk A, Pierzchala W, Sozanska E. Interleukin-17 in sputum correlates with airway hyper-responsiveness to methacholine. Respir Med. 2003;97(6):726–33.
41. Chatenoud L. Natural and induced T CD4+CD25+FOXP3+ regulatory T cells. Methods Mol Biol. 2011;677:3–13. https://doi.org/10.1007/978-1-60761-869-0_1.
42. Shevach EM. Mechanisms of foxp3+ T regulatory cell-mediated suppression. Immunity. 2009;30(5):636–45. https://doi.org/10.1016/j.immuni.2009.04.010.
43. Sakaguchi S, Wing K, Onishi Y, Prieto-Martin P, Yamaguchi T. Regulatory T cells: how do they suppress immune responses? Int Immunol. 2009;21(10):1105–11. https://doi.org/10.1093/intimm/dxp095.
44. Akdis M, Verhagen J, Taylor A, Karamloo F, Karagiannidis C, Crameri R, et al. Immune responses in healthy and allergic individuals are characterized by a fine balance between allergen-specific T regulatory 1 and T helper 2 cells. J Exp Med. 2004;199(11):1567–75. https://doi.org/10.1084/jem.20032058.
45. Hartl D, Koller B, Mehlhorn AT, Reinhardt D, Nicolai T, Schendel DJ, et al. Quantitative and functional impairment of pulmonary CD4+CD25hi regulatory T cells in pediatric asthma. J Allergy Clin Immunol. 2007;119(5):1258–66. https://doi.org/10.1016/j.jaci.2007.02.023.
46. Spits H, Di Santo JP. The expanding family of innate lymphoid cells: regulators and effectors of immunity and tissue remodeling. Nat Immunol. 2011;12(1):21–7. https://doi.org/10.1038/ni.1962.

47. Wilhelm C, Hirota K, Stieglitz B, Van Snick J, Tolaini M, Lahl K, et al. An IL-9 fate reporter demonstrates the induction of an innate IL-9 response in lung inflammation. Nat Immunol. 2011;12(11):1071–7. https://doi.org/10.1038/ni.2133.
48. Constantinides MG, McDonald BD, Verhoef PA, Bendelac A. A committed precursor to innate lymphoid cells. Nature. 2014;508(7496):397–401. https://doi.org/10.1038/nature13047.
49. Mjosberg J, Bernink J, Golebski K, Karrich JJ, Peters CP, Blom B, et al. The transcription factor GATA3 is essential for the function of human type 2 innate lymphoid cells. Immunity. 2012;37(4):649–59. https://doi.org/10.1016/j.immuni.2012.08.015.
50. Klein Wolterink RG, Kleinjan A, van Nimwegen M, Bergen I, de Bruijn M, Levani Y, et al. Pulmonary innate lymphoid cells are major producers of IL-5 and IL-13 in murine models of allergic asthma. Eur J Immunol. 2012;42(5):1106–16. https://doi.org/10.1002/eji.201142018.
51. Smith SG, Chen R, Kjarsgaard M, Huang C, Oliveria JP, O'Byrne PM, et al. Increased numbers of activated group 2 innate lymphoid cells in the airways of patients with severe asthma and persistent airway eosinophilia. J Allergy Clin Immunol. 2016;137(1):75–86.e8. https://doi.org/10.1016/j.jaci.2015.05.037.
52. Drake LY, Iijima K, Kita H. Group 2 innate lymphoid cells and CD4+ T cells cooperate to mediate type 2 immune response in mice. Allergy. 2014;69(10):1300–7. https://doi.org/10.1111/all.12446.
53. Mirchandani AS, Besnard AG, Yip E, Scott C, Bain CC, Cerovic V, et al. Type 2 innate lymphoid cells drive CD4+ Th2 cell responses. J Immunol. 2014;192(5):2442–8. https://doi.org/10.4049/jimmunol.1300974.
54. Kabata H, Moro K, Fukunaga K, Suzuki Y, Miyata J, Masaki K, et al. Thymic stromal lymphopoietin induces corticosteroid resistance in natural helper cells during airway inflammation. Nat Commun. 2013;4:2675. https://doi.org/10.1038/ncomms3675.

Chapter 4
Mechanisms for Non-eosinophilic Asthma

Arihiko Kanehiro

Abstract Asthma can be broadly subdivided into eosinophilic or non-eosinophilic phenotypes based on the inflammatory cellular patterns seen in sputum, blood, and airway tissue. However, the most appropriate cutoff value of non-eosinophilic asthma that identifies individuals in whom neutrophils are activated and contributing to the pathogenic processes in asthma is not elucidated compared to eosinophilic asthma. Major clinical phenotypes of non-eosinophilic asthma include those patients with neutrophilic, paucigranulocytic, and late-onset obesity-related asthma. The mechanism of non-eosinophilic asthma is very complicated and has not been investigated in detail; nonetheless many potential molecular pathways may be implicated in the development of non-eosinophilic asthma.

The cause of airway neutrophilia in asthma is possibly due to augmented innate immunity, IL-23-Th17-IL-17-ILC3 pathway-mediated neutrophilic inflammation, delayed apoptosis of neutrophils caused by epithelial cell-derived cytokines and growth factors, corticosteroid treatment inducing impaired apoptosis of neutrophils, and ineffective macrophage efferocytosis of neutrophils, upregulated NLRP-3 inflammasome and p38/MAPK activity, and reduced lipoxin levels, as well as an altered airway microbiome. Non-eosinophilic inflammation is associated with an impaired therapeutic response to inhaled corticosteroids and usually results in severe uncontrolled asthma. Better understanding of the mechanisms of non-eosinophilic inflammation in asthma will identify new approaches for the treatment of severe non-eosinophilic asthma patients.

A. Kanehiro (✉)
Department of Internal Medicine, Allergy and Respiratory Center, Okayama Rosai Hospital, Okayama, Japan
e-mail: akanehir@md.okayama-u.ac.jp

A. Yokoyama (ed.), *Advances in Asthma*, Respiratory Disease Series: Diagnostic Tools and Disease Managements, https://doi.org/10.1007/978-981-13-2790-2_4

Keywords Eosinophilic asthma · Non-eosinophilic asthma · Non-eosinophilic airway inflammation · Neutrophilic inflammation · Paucigranulocytic inflammation

Abbreviations

CXCL1	Chemokine ligand 1
CXCR2	Chemokine receptor 2
Cys-LTs	Cysteinyl leukotrienes
ECP	Eosinophil cationic protein
EPO	Eosinophil peroxidase
IFN	Interferon
ILC	Innate lymphoid cell
LT	Leukotriene
MBP	Major basic protein
MMP-9	Matrix metalloproteinase-9
NK cell	Natural killer cell
NKT cell	Natural killer T cell
PGD2	Prostaglandin D2
ROS	Reactive oxygen species
TGF-β	Transforming growth factor-β
TNF-α	Tumor necrosis factor-α
TSLP	Thymic stromal lymphopoietin

4.1 Introduction

Asthma can be subdivided into "eosinophilic (type 2 adaptive immune response and innate immune response)" or "non-eosinophilic (non-type 2)" phenotypes based on the inflammatory cellular patterns seen in the sputum, blood, and airway tissue. Non-eosinophilic airway inflammation is a term used to describe a subtype of asthma associated with normal numbers of sputum eosinophils. Up to 50% of never smokers or ex-smoker patients with stable mild to severe asthma have non-eosinophilic inflammation, and this inflammatory phenotype is also found in smokers with asthma, some patients with a high body mass index (BMI), or occupational asthma. The non-eosinophilic phenotype is typically subdivided into neutrophilic inflammation when neutrophil numbers are raised above a defined cutoff level or paucigranulocytic inflammation when both eosinophil and neutrophil numbers are normal. The relative proportion of each subtype is uncertain because of variable cutoff points used to define neutrophilia. Moreover, the most appropriate value that indicates whether neutrophils are activated and contributing to the pathogenic processes in asthma is unclarified. The urgent development of novel therapies is essential in non-eosinophilic phenotypes such as neutrophilic or paucigranulocytic asthma, where no targeted biologic or other new therapies are yet available and outcomes of studies are still lacking because of no good biomarkers in non-eosinophilic asthma.

4.2 Cellular Profiles of Eosinophilic and Non-eosinophilic Asthma

Sputum cellular profiles are believed to directly reflect lung inflammation and are the preferred method used in asthma research to determine eosinophilic asthma. Sputum cutoff eosinophil levels of greater than 2–3% have been used to define eosinophilic asthma. Technical requirements for sputum processing and cell counting may limit the feasibility of using sputum eosinophil counts in all clinics and hospitals, and furthermore, bronchial wall biopsy samples must be obtained by bronchoscopy which is not routinely performed in asthmatics outside of the research setting specialized hospitals. However, sputum eosinophil counts are associated with bronchial tissue eosinophil numbers suggesting that they provide a good indicator of airway eosinophilic pathology [1]. In contrast, the cutoff for an elevated sputum neutrophil count is not clearly established with range from as low as >40% to as high as ≥76% reported in the literature. The most appropriate cutoff value that identifies individuals in whom neutrophils are activated and contributing to the pathogenic processes in asthma is not elucidated. In addition, sputum neutrophils do not correlate with bronchial tissue numbers, bringing into query their predictive value for identifying neutrophil-induced airway inflammation [1]. Additionally, blood neutrophil levels have not been strongly correlated with airway neutrophil counts and other reliable biomarkers of airway neutrophilia have not yet been established [2].

4.3 Clinical Characteristics of Non-eosinophilic Asthma

The endotypes associated with clinical phenotypes characterized by eosinophilia include early-onset allergic asthma, late-onset eosinophilic asthma, aspirin-exacerbated respiratory disease (AERD), allergic bronchopulmonary mycosis (ABPM), and exercise-induced asthma (EIA). On the other hand, non-eosinophilic inflammation occurs clinically in approximately 50% of never smokers or ex-smokers with mild to severe asthma and is commonly found in current smokers with asthma, with or without neutrophilic inflammation [3]. Patients with neutrophilic asthma develop at an older age and less atopic and demonstrate fixed airflow obstruction and corticosteroid insensitivity. Clinical characteristics of paucigranulocytic asthma are late (adult) onset and less atopic, and both eosinophil and

	Clinical	Pathobiology
Early-onset allergic Childhood onset Long standing asthma	Aeroallergen sensitivity Other allergic diseases	Th2 cytokines IgE-mediated Eosinophil less clear in severe disease
Persistent eosinophilic Late(adult) onset, often severe	Sinusitis, Nasal polyps Less atopic	Blood and lung eosinophils ILC2 immunity
Aspirin-exacerbated respiratory disease Adult onset, often severe Predominantly female	Sinusitis, Nasal polyps Less atopic Bronchospasm with NSAID/aspirin	CysLTs pathway
Allergic bronchopulmonary mycosis Late (adult) onset, often severe	Increased cough/mucus Central bronchiectasis	Blood and lung eosinophils, High IgE Mixed adaptive immunity Fungal colonization
Obesity-related Late (adult) onset Predominantly female	Very symptomatic Less airflow obstruction Less atopic	Neutrophilic or paucigranulocytic IL-17-ILC3 axis
Paucigranulocytic Late (adult) onset Mild and severe	Fixed airflow obstruction Less atopic Corticosteroid insensitivity	Paucigranulocytic Subepithelial fibrosis Smooth muscle hypertrophy
Neutrophilic Late (adult) onset	Fixed airflow obstruction Less atopic Smoking history Corticosteroid insensitivity	Neutrophils IL-23-Th17-IL-17 axis Augmented innate immunity Inflammasome

Fig. 4.1 Phenotypes in relation to eosinophilic or non-eosinophilic inflammation

neutrophil numbers are normal and indicate fixed airflow obstruction because of airway smooth muscle hypertrophy and subepithelial fibrosis. High BMI severe asthma is late (adult) onset and predominantly female and very symptomatic but with less airflow obstruction and usually associated with non-eosinophilic or paucigranulocytic phenotype, while others have submucosal eosinophilia [4]. Taken together, clinical phenotypes of asthma not associated with eosinophils (non-eosinophilic phenotypes) include those patients with neutrophilic asthma, asthma with fixed airflow obstruction and very little inflammation (paucigranulocytic), and late-onset obesity-related asthma (Fig. 4.1). Other non-eosinophilic clinical phenotypes that endotypes are still less defined include occupational asthma due to low molecular weight agents or environmental pollution, and respiratory infections. In general, non-eosinophilic inflammation is associated with an impaired therapeutic response to inhaled corticosteroids, although the detailed pathobiologic pathways are not yet defined [5].

4.4 Evidence for Neutrophil Activation in Asthma

Recent many evidences suggest that innate immune system is activated in chronic asthma. Sputum IL-8 and neutrophil elastase concentrations and innate immune receptors-Toll-like receptors (TLR) 2, TLR4, and cluster of differentiation (CD) 14 as well as pro-inflammatory IL-8 and IL-1β gene expression levels are increased in neutrophilic asthma compared to non-neutrophilic asthma [6]. Neutrophil activation, as measured by sputum myeloperoxidase (MPO) levels in asthmatics, is positively associated with sputum neutrophil numbers. Furthermore, specific sputum gene expression signatures are reported to discriminate eosinophilic asthma from non-eosinophilic asthma as well as to predict a beneficial response to inhaled corticosteroids [7]. Non-eosinophilic asthma was identified by increased sputum cell expression of IL-1β, alkaline phosphatase tissue-nonspecific isozyme (ALPL), and CXCR2, whereas eosinophilic asthma was characterized by increased expression of galectin-10 (CLC), carboxypeptidase A3 (CPA3), and deoxyribonuclease I-like 3 (DNASE1L3). The nucleotide-binding domain, leucine-rich repeat-containing family protein (NLRP)-3 inflammasome is upregulated in neutrophilic asthma and may increase the production of IL-1β [8]. Anti-inflammatory responses may be impaired in non-eosinophilic asthma based on reduced sputum galectin-3 concentrations, which increases uptake of apoptotic neutrophils and reduced IL-1RA/IL-1β ratio and which might increase pro-inflammatory actions of IL-1β [9]. Soluble receptor for advanced glycation end products (RAGE) is deficient in bronchoalveolar lavage (BAL) samples in neutrophilic asthma. T-cell granzyme B pathway, which is thought to mediate apoptosis of epithelial cells, might be defective in non-eosinophilic asthma, based on the finding of a higher ratio of the expression of granzyme B to its inhibitor in T cells in this group compared to eosinophilic asthma [10].

In addition, systemic inflammation is increased in patients with neutrophilic airway inflammation. The proportion of patients with elevated CRP, IL-6, and neutrophil elastase concentrations is higher in neutrophilic asthma compared to a non-neutrophilic group. Neutrophilic inflammation is associated with increased α-defensin and neutrophil protease gene expression in blood [11]. In non-eosinophilic asthma, blood neutrophils released significantly higher levels of IL-8 at rest [11]. Furthermore, gene expression markers of systemic inflammation were associated with higher BMI, heavy history of cigarette smoking, lower predicted forced vital capacity (FVC), and increased sputum neutrophils [12].

4.5 Mechanisms of Eosinophilic and Non-eosinophilic Asthma

Compared to eosinophilic asthma, which type 2 adaptive immune response and innate immune response play an important role, mechanism of non-eosinophilic asthma is very complicated and has not been investigated in detail. In major subphenotypes of non-eosinophilic asthma including neutrophilic asthma, paucigranulocytic asthma, and obesity-related asthma, many potential molecular pathways may be implicated in the development of non-eosinophilic asthma independent of corticosteroid use (Figs. 4.1 and 4.2).

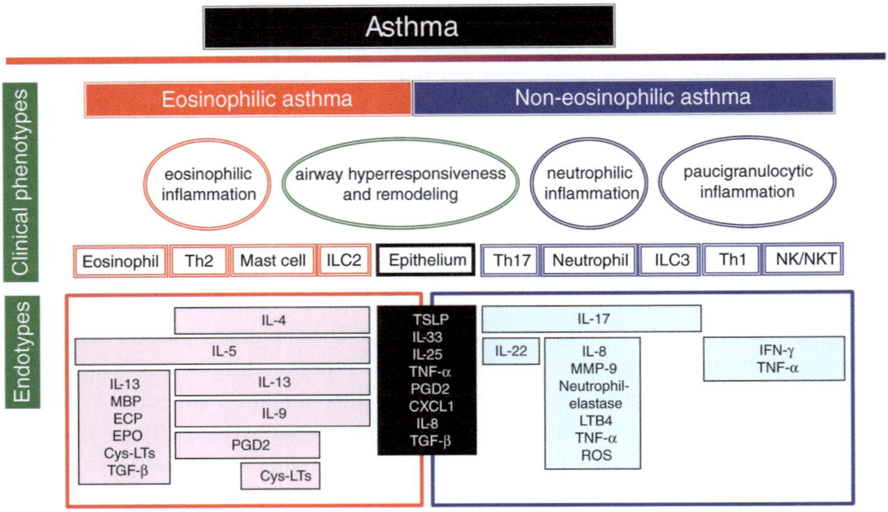

Fig. 4.2 Asthma phenotypes and endotypes of eosinophilic or non-eosinophilic asthma

4.5.1 Mechanisms of Neutrophilic Asthma

Clinically, patients with neutrophilic asthma develop at an older age and demonstrate impaired lung function, less bronchodilator reversibility, and less atopy. However, detailed mechanisms of neutrophilic asthma are not well-defined. Corticosteroids are known to inhibit neutrophil apoptosis, which in turn may prolong or promote airway neutrophilia, potentially contributing to the diagnosis of neutrophilic asthma. A significant proportion of patients with asthma are current smokers, at rates similar to the general population. Multiple cohorts have described smokers with asthma as suffering from more severe disease and having fewer sputum eosinophils; ex-smokers and current smokers have predominant neutrophilic inflammation [3]. Steroid insensitivity in this phenotype may be due to alterations in histone deacetylase activity. Cigarette smoke is toxic to the respiratory epithelium and may induce type 2 inflammation from the subepithelial dendritic cells. Occupational asthma due to low-molecular-weight agents and secondary to environmental pollution may be induced by similar pathways.

IL-23 leads to neutrophil infiltration in the airway of asthmatic mice, which is characteristic of severe asthma resulting from Th17 development and subsequently IL-17 secretion.

Th17 inflammation is related to a severe phenotype, frequent exacerbations, steroid resistance, bronchial wall remodeling, mucus hypersecretion, and smooth muscle hypertrophy [13, 14]. IL-17 can induce prominent neutrophilic inflammation and the IL-23-Th17-IL-17 axis is gaining significant attention for its contribution to both neutrophilic and mixed granulocytic airway inflammation. IL-23 leads to neutrophilic infiltration in the airway of asthmatic mice, which is characteristic of severe asthma resulting from Th17 development and subsequently IL-17 secretion.

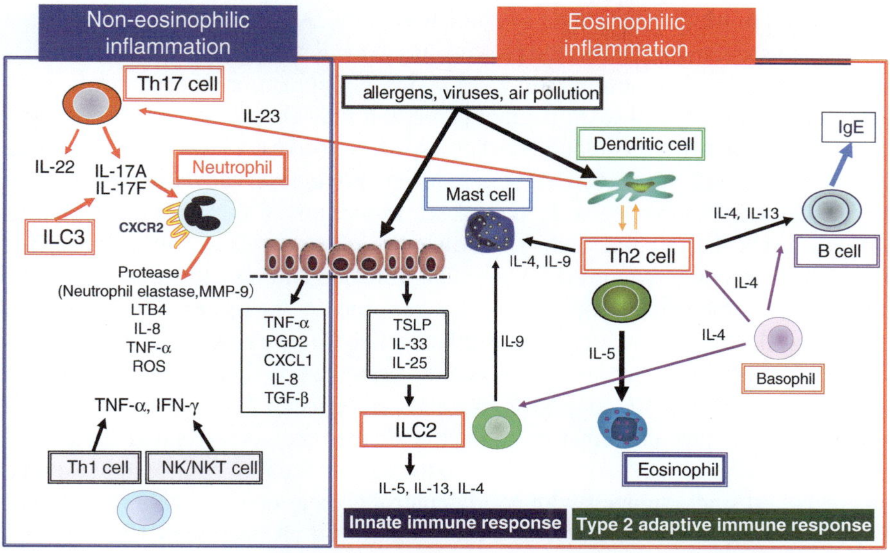

Fig. 4.3 Mechanisms of eosinophilic and non-eosinophilic inflammation in asthma

IL-17 may also contribute to severe asthma by inducing relative steroid unresponsiveness [15] (Fig. 4.3). In neutrophilic asthma, there is evidence of upregulated NLRP-3 inflammasome activity [16]. In a recent study using transcriptome-associated clusters, the cluster which was characterized by IFN-, TNF-, and inflammasome-associated genes had the greatest sputum neutrophilia as compared with other clusters which were associated with type 2 inflammation or metabolic/mitochondrial genes and sputum eosinophilia [17]. This suggests a role for inflammasome mechanisms in neutrophilic asthma. Airway inflammations through both the acquired and innate immune pathways may distinguish neutrophilic asthma from eosinophilic asthma. The innate immune response is activated during infection (viral, bacterial) or during irritant environmental exposure, such as endotoxin, ozone, and fine particulate matter exposures. Instead of triggering ILC2 or Th2 pathways, these agents can activate TLR4 and CD14 on epithelial cells and macrophages leading to nuclear factor (NF)-κB activation, which in turn establishes a highly pro-inflammatory condition [6]. This leads to amplified production of IL-8 which recruits activated neutrophils into the airways.

Another important pathway for an increase in sputum neutrophil levels in neutrophilic asthma may be the result of impaired alveolar macrophage phagocytosis of apoptotic cells (efferocytosis). In a study of patients with stable asthma undergoing sputum induction, macrophage efferocytosis was impaired in patients with neutrophilic asthma, leading to persistent airway neutrophilia, but was not impaired in those with eosinophilic asthma [18]. p38 kinase, which is the mitogen-activated protein kinase (MAPK) family, is induced by environmental triggers (e.g., endotoxin, oxidative stress, cigarette smoke, air pollution) relevant to asthma and specifically to non-eosinophilic asthma. Inhibition of p38/MAPK mitigates neutrophilic inflammation, which may play a role in neutrophilic asthma [19]. The lipoxins are endogenous arachidonate-derived pro-resolution mediators that decrease inflammation and are reduced in severe asthma. Lipoxins inhibit neutrophil chemotaxis, transcellular migration, and toxic degranulation and may support natural killer (NK) cell function as well as eosinophil trafficking in severe asthma [20]. Oxidative stress in asthmatic airways is associated with reduced lipoxin levels and also with activity of the enzyme-soluble epoxide hydrolase. Inhibition of this enzyme increases lipoxin levels that mediate anti-inflammatory pathways relevant to asthma [21]. CC16 has been directly correlated with lung function and may function as an anti-inflammatory mediator through effects at the lipoxin A4 receptor which is also expressed ILC2 [22]. Treatments that enhance lipoxin levels or CC16 may be beneficial in neutrophilic asthma, performed the prominent cellular effects of lipoxins on lung neutrophils. NK and NKT-like cells are effector lymphocytes that are a major source of pro-inflammatory and cytotoxic mediators with relative corticosteroid insensitivity which may contribute to the development of neutrophilic asthma. In one cohort study, subjects with poorly controlled neutrophilic asthma had higher expression of granzyme B by $CD8^{+}$ T cells, high IFN-γ production by NK cells, and greater TNF-α production by NKT-like cells than healthy control subjects [23]. Cytotoxic effects of granzyme B may lead to increased epithelial cell death and chronic inflammation, which contribute to persistent symptoms despite corticosteroids therapy. Chronic infection may be a key underlying stimulus for this Th17-type inflammatory response in asthma, given that Th17 cells produce IL-17 in addition to other pro-inflammatory cytokines in response to bacterial and fungal infection. There is evidence suggesting that 15-lipoxygenase metabolites such as 15-hydroxyeicosatetraenoic acid are important mediators in the development of Th1 inflammation induced by ovalbumin and double-stranded RNA in a murine model of asthma. This suggests that neutrophilic asthma could be a manifestation of asthmatics with underlying chronic subclinical infection or inhaled exposures [24]. Virus-associated neutrophilic asthma with high IFN-γ, an exacerbation-prone clinical phenotype, may be explained by a Th1 response via a 15-lipoxygenase mechanism [25].

4.5.2 Mechanisms of Paucigranulocytic Asthma

Paucigranulocytic asthma represents up to 40% of non-eosinophilic asthma [26]. Although paucigranulocytic asthma is associated with well-controlled or mild intermittent asthma in the SARP cohort, it can be severe and may not respond well to standard asthma medications such as inhaled corticosteroids. The mechanisms underlying paucigranulocytic asthma are believed to be related to abnormalities or dysfunction of structural cells, including airway smooth muscle, nerves, and vascular tissue. Airway remodeling, such as airway smooth muscle hypertrophy, subepithelial fibrosis, and mucus gland hypertrophy, may occur as a result of aberrant repair mechanisms. Moreover, airway bronchospasm can induce transforming growth factor-β (TGF-β) release and subepithelial fibrosis in the airway. Hence in paucigranulocytic asthma, this abnormal airway smooth muscle can not only contract to cause severe airflow obstruction but also actively secrete chemokines and cytokines that promote and mediate inflammation.

4.5.3 *Mechanisms of Obesity-Related Non-eosinophilic Asthma*

Obesity is increasingly recognized as important and consistent variables in the development and severity of asthma. Obesity-related asthma in a late-onset, female-dominant phenotype is associated with neutrophilic or paucigranulocytic airway inflammation with low eosinophil counts. In these patients, peripheral lung tissue elastance and airway resistance are abnormally elevated; nevertheless the increased peripheral airway hyperresponsiveness can be reversed with significant weight loss [27, 28]. The mechanisms underlying these changes may relate to inflammation in the adipose tissue mediated by activated macrophages, causing increases in IL-6, TNF-α, and leptin that are also reversible with weight loss. Patients with obesity-related asthma may be more sensitive to environmental pollutants and irritants compared to nonobese asthma. Ozone exposure can decrease lung function, increase airway neutrophilia, and induce IL-6 in obese female asthma. In a high-fat diet mouse model of obese asthma, airway hyperreactivity was found to be independent of adaptive immunity and instead characterized by IL-17A released by ILC3 cells and macrophage-derived IL-1β [29]. Consumption of a low antioxidant diet is associated with progression of asthma symptoms, reduced lung function, and increased percentage of sputum neutrophils. Obesity is a complex modulator of inflammation that affects not only eosinophilic asthma by perpetuating Type2/Th2 inflammation but also non-eosinophilic asthma as a distinct subphenotype driven by several mechanisms or endotypes.

4.6 Implications for the Treatment of Non-eosinophilic Asthma

The mainstay of asthma treatment is inhaled corticosteroids, although clinical evidence indicates that non-eosinophilic asthma is generally poorly responsive to corticosteroid treatment in both symptoms and lung function, and, furthermore, corticosteroid treatment could potentially worsen the disease in some asthma patients. There is a critical unmet need for novel treatments that will impact on clinical outcomes in severe asthma patients with non-eosinophilic inflammation. Non-pharmacologic prevention and treatment of non-eosinophilic asthma include smoking cessation, avoidance of environmental and occupational pollutants, dietary changes, and treatment of comorbid conditions that could lead to neutrophilic asthma, such as infection and obesity. Off-label use of medications such as macrolide antibiotics or statins in non-eosinophilic asthma appears to have limited or selective efficacy, and currently they lack the clinical data to support their extensive use in non-eosinophilic asthma. Recently, targeting the structural airway cells such as bronchial thermoplasty may prove to be useful in paucigranulocytic asthma or obesity-related asthma. Additional studies are needed to evaluate the effect of novel small-molecule inhibitors and biologic agents that can be targeted to treat non-eosinophilic asthma.

4.7 Conclusions

Uncover new knowledge about the mechanisms and molecular phenotypes underlying the endotypes for non-eosinophilic asthma as well as eosinophilic asthma is an urgent need. We have to settle this phenotyping with the more descriptive cytokine-based or endotypic nomenclature. Non-eosinophilic inflammation is associated with an impaired therapeutic response to inhaled corticosteroids. Neutrophilic inflammation is associated with activation of the innate immune system in asthma and systemic inflammation. Several mechanisms either alone or in combination could explain elevated sputum neutrophil counts in asthma including corticosteroids, associated chronic sino-bronchopulmonary infection, delayed human neutrophil apoptosis due to epithelial cell-derived cytokines and growth factors, impaired macrophage phagocytosis, and an altered airway microbiome. Taken together, the finding suggests that non-eosinophilic inflammation and Th2-low inflammation in nonsmokers with asthma share some similar immunopathological features, including normal eosinophil numbers, submucosal mast cell numbers, and subepithelial basement membrane thickness. Due to the lack of effective specific therapies targeting non-eosinophilic inflammation including neutrophilic inflammation, there is currently no definitive evidence for the involvement of these inflammatory phenotypes in chronic asthma. Additional pathways may account for poor asthma control in patients with non-eosinophilic asthma including Th1 inflammation, Th17 inflammation, or a combination of Th2 and Th17 inflammation, as well as corticosteroid insensitivity. Non-inflammatory mechanisms may also be important in some individuals including fixed airway hyperresponsiveness and airway remodeling.

There is an unmet need for novel treatments that will impact on clinical outcomes in patients with non-eosinophilic inflammation. Development of biological agents to target non-eosinophilic inflammation in asthma has been disappointing to date with the termination of clinical studies of monoclonal antibodies targeting IL-17 and TNF-α. In the near future, the selection of patients with severe asthma and evidence of Th17 high inflammation may be more likely to identify a subpopulation respond to IL-17 blockers. Currently, long-acting muscarinic antagonist (LAMA) or bronchial thermoplasty are possible treatment options for symptomatic patients with paucigranulocytic inflammation in whom there is no evidence of activated inflammatory pathways or corticosteroid insensitivity that could be targeted by specific therapies. Better understanding of the mechanisms of non-eosinophilic inflammation in asthma will identify new approaches for the treatment of severe non-eosinophilic asthma.

References

1. Arron J, Choy D, Laviolette M, Kelsen S, Hatab A, Leigh R. Disconnect between sputum neutrophils and other measures of airway inflammation in asthma. Eur Respir J. 2014;43:627–9.
2. Hastie AT, Moore WC, Li H, Rector BM, Ortega VE, Pascual RM, National Heart, Lung, and Blood Institute's Severe Asthma Research Program, et al. Biomarker surrogates do not accurately predict sputum eosinophil and neutrophil percentages in asthmatic subjects. J Allergy Clin Immunol. 2013;132:72–80.
3. Thomson NC, Chaudhuri R, Heaney L, Bucknall C, Niven R, Brightling C. Clinical outcomes and inflammatory biomarkers in current smokers and exsmokers with severe asthma. J Allergy Clin Immunol. 2013;131:1008–16.
4. Desai D, Newby C, Symon F, Haldar P, Shah S, Gupta S. Elevated sputum interleukin-5 and submucosal eosinophilia in obese individuals with severe asthma. Am J Respir Crit Care Med. 2013;188:657–63.
5. McGrath K, Icitovic N, Boushey H, Lazarus S, Sutherland E, Chinchilli V. A large subgroup of mild-to-moderate asthma is persistently noneosinophilic. Am J Respir Crit Care Med. 2012;185:612–9.
6. Wood L, Baines K, Fu J, Scott H, Gibson P. The neutrophilic inflammatory phenotype is associated with systemic inflammation in asthma. Chest. 2012;142:86–93.
7. Baines K, Simpson J, Wood L, Scott R, Fibbens N, Powell H. Sputum gene expression signature of 6 biomarkers discriminates asthma inflammatory phenotypes. J Allergy Clin Immunol. 2014;133:997–1007.
8. Simpson J, Phipps S, Baines K, Oreo K, Gunawardhana L, Gibson P. Elevated expression of the NLRP3 inflammasome in neutrophilic asthma. Eur Respir J. 2014;43:1067–76.
9. Gao P, Gibson P, Baines K, Yang I, Upham J, Reynolds P. Anti-inflammatory deficiencies in neutrophilic asthma: reduced galectin-3 and IL-1RA/IL-1β. Respir Res. 2015;16:5.
10. Simpson J, Gibson P, Yang I, Upham J, James A, Reynolds P, et al. Altered sputum granzyme B and granzyme B/proteinase inhibitor-9 in patients with noneosinophilic asthma. Respirology. 2014;19:280–7.
11. Baines K, Simpson J, Bowden N, Scott R, Gibson P. Differential gene expression and cytokine production from neutrophils in asthma phenotypes. Eur Respir J. 2010;35:522–31.
12. Fu J, Baines K, Wood L, Gibson P. Systemic inflammation is associated with differential gene expression and airway neutrophilia in asthma. OMICS. 2013;17:187–99.
13. Cosmi L, Liotta F, Annunziato F. Th17 regulating lower airway disease. Curr Opin Allergy Clin Immunol. 2016;16:1–6.
14. Ricciardolo FLM, Sorbello V, Folino A, Gallo F, Massaglia GM, Favatà G, et al. Identification of IL-17F/frequent exacerbator endotype in asthma. J Allergy Clin Immunol. 2017;140:395–406.
15. McKinley L, Alcorn JF, Peterson A, Dupont RB, Kapadia S, Logar A, et al. TH17 cells mediate steroid-resistant airway inflammation and airway hyperresponsiveness in mice. J Immunol. 2008;181:4089–97.
16. Kim RY, Pinkerton JW, Essilfie AT, Robertson AAB, Baines KJ, Brown AC, et al. Role for NLRP3 inflammasome-mediated, IL-1β-dependent responses in severe, steroid-resistant asthma. Am J Respir Crit Care Med. 2017;196:283–97.
17. Kuo CS, Pavlidis S, Loza M, Baribaud F, Rowe A, Pandis I, et al. U-BIOPRED Study group. T-helper cell type 2 (Th2) and non-Th2 molecular phenotypes of asthma using sputum transcriptomics in U-BIOPRED. Eur Respir J. 2017;49:1602135. https://doi.org/10.1183/13993003.02135-2016.

18. Simpson JL, Gibson PG, Yang IA, Upham J, James A, Reynolds PN, AMAZES Study Research Group, et al. Impaired macrophage phagocytosis in non-eosinophilic asthma. Clin Exp Allergy. 2013;43:29–35.
19. Chung KF. p38 mitogen-activated protein kinase pathways in asthma and COPD. Chest. 2011;139:1470–9.
20. Duvall MG, Barnig C, Cernadas M, Ricklefs I, Krishnamoorthy N, Grossman NL, National Heart Lung, and Blood Institute's Severe Asthma Research Program-3 Investigators, et al. Natural killer cell-mediated inflammation resolution is disabled in severe asthma. Sci Immunol. 2017;2:eaam5446. https://doi.org/10.1126/sciimmunol.aam5446.
21. Ono E, Dutile S, Kazani S, Wechsler ME, Yang J, Hammock BD, National Heart, Lung, and Blood Institute's Asthma Clinical Research Network, et al. Lipoxin generation is related to soluble epoxide hydrolase activity in severe asthma. Am J Respir Crit Care Med. 2014;190:886–97.
22. Guerra S, Halonen M, Vasquez MM, Spangenberg A, Stern DA, Morgan WJ, et al. Relation between circulating CC16 concentrations, lung function, and development of chronic obstructive pulmonary disease across the lifespan: a prospective study. Lancet Respir Med. 2015;3:613–20.
23. Hodge S, Hodge G, Simpson JL, Yang IA, Upham J, James A, AMAZES Study Research Group, et al. Blood cytotoxic/inflammatory mediators in non-eosinophilic asthma. Clin Exp Allergy. 2016;46:60–70.
24. Kim YS, Choi JP, Kim MH, Park HK, Yang S, Kim YS, et al. IgG sensitization to extracellular vesicles in indoor dust is closely associated with the prevalence of non-eosinophilic asthma, COPD, and lung cancer. Allergy, Asthma Immunol Res. 2016;8:198–205.
25. Jeon SG, Moon HG, Kim YS, Choi JP, Shin TS, Hong SW, et al. 15-lipoxygenase metabolites play an important role in the development of a T-helper type 1 allergic inflammation induced by double-stranded RNA. Clin Exp Allergy. 2009;39:908–17.
26. Demarche S, Schleich F, Henket M, Paulus V, Van Hees T, Louis R. Detailed analysis of sputum and systemic inflammation in asthma phenotypes: are paucigranulocytic asthmatics really non-inflammatory? BMC Pulm Med. 2016;16:46.
27. Al-Alwan A, Bates JH, Chapman DG, Kaminsky DA, DeSarno MJ, Irvin CG, et al. The nonallergic asthma of obesity: a matter of distal lung compliance. Am J Respir Crit Care Med. 2014;189:1494–502.
28. Ather JL, Chung M, Hoyt LR, Randall MJ, Georgsdottir A, Daphtary NA, et al. Weight loss decreases inherent and allergic methacholine hyperresponsiveness in mouse models of diet-induced obese asthma. Am J Respir Cell Mol Biol. 2016;55:176–87.
29. Kim HY, Lee HJ, Chang YJ, Pichavant M, Shore SA, Fitzgerald KA, et al. Interleukin-17-producing innate lymphoid cells and the NLRP3 inflammasome facilitate obesity-associated airway hyperreactivity. Nat Med. 2014;20:54–61.

Chapter 5
Corticosteroid Resistance in Asthma

Koichi Fukunaga

Abstract Although inhaled corticosteroid (ICS) is the typical medication for the treatment of asthma worldwide, there are patients who are nonresponsive to the treatment. Patients with GC-resistant asthma show more frequent exacerbation than other asthmatics, and the number of clinical consultations is much higher. It has been recognized in recent years that asthma is not a single disease; it is a syndrome with various phenotypes. The heterogeneity complicates the analysis of the pathology associated with GC resistance. However, the characterization of the inflammatory and immunological phenotypes and the classification into several end types will be crucial for elucidating the mechanism of GC-resistant asthma. Future work on the molecular mechanisms of GC resistance will facilitate the selection of therapeutic drugs according to the pathology of individual patients with refractory asthma resistant to GC treatment.

Keywords Asthma · Steroid resistant · Type 2 innate lymphoid cell · Th17 cell

5.1 Introduction

The widespread use of inhaled corticosteroids (ICS) as first-line drugs for the treatment of asthma is linked to a decline in asthma-related deaths. However, there are some patients in whom asthma cannot be controlled by using ICS because of genetic predispositions, dysfunction of the glucocorticoid receptor, modifications in inflammatory cells, comorbidities such as sinusitis and obesity, and poor adherence to

K. Fukunaga (✉)
Pulmonary Division, Department of Medicine, Keio University School of Medicine, Tokyo, Japan
e-mail: km-fuku@cpnet.med.keio.ac.jp

A. Yokoyama (ed.), *Advances in Asthma*, Respiratory Disease Series: Diagnostic Tools and Disease Managements, https://doi.org/10.1007/978-981-13-2790-2_5

therapy. Here, we review our current knowledge about the resistance mechanism against corticosteroids, also known as glucocorticoids (GC).

5.2 Mechanism of GC Action

The mechanism of GC action depends on the activation of intracellular GC receptor (GR) molecules (Fig. 5.1). Alternative splicing of the *GR* primary transcript generates two isoforms, GRα and GRβ. GRα is present in all organs and tissues and primarily found in the cytoplasm associated with heat shock protein (HSP) 90 and other regulatory molecules. When GC passes through the cell membrane and binds to GRα, it causes the dissociation of HSP90 and the other molecules and facilitates the translocation into the nucleus. The GC-GRα complex forms a homodimer in the nucleus and binds to various gene promoter regions called GC-responsive elements (GRE), which induce or suppress gene transcription. Typically, nuclear factor (NF)-κB and activator protein (AP)-1 activate transcription of various inflammatory genes (cytokines, chemokines, among others), but the GC-GRα complex activity mediated by a corepressor molecule suppresses both transcription activators. In addition, the GC-GRα complex induces histone deacetylase (HDAC) 2, which aggregates chromatin structure by deacetylating histones, functioning as a transcriptional suppressor of induced inflammatory genes [1].

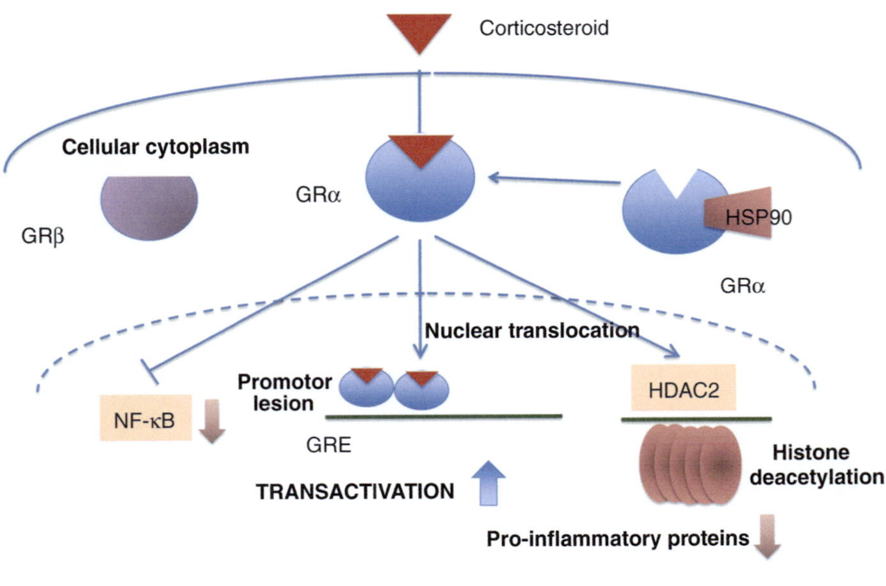

Fig. 5.1 The mechanism of GC action

5.3 Definition of GC Resistance in Clinical Practice

Less than 15% of asthma patients but approximately 30% of patients with severe asthma experience GC-refractory disease, despite combinatorial treatment with high dose of ICS. The definition of airflow limitation is observed after bronchodilator administration, but >15% improvement in the forced expiratory volume in 1 second (FEV1) cannot be achieved even if a systemic GC (e.g., prednisolone 40 mg) is administered for 14 days [2, 3]. Moreover, recent reports indicated that sensitivity to GC did not clinically improve even if the number of eosinophils in the sputum and the FEV1 were partially improved by systemic GC drug administration [4]. In clinical practice, GC resistance has to be considered if symptom control is insufficient even when using medium to high doses of ICS (fluticasone propionate, ≥500 μg, or budesonide, ≥800 μg) in combination with long-acting beta-2 agonists, leukotriene receptor antagonists, and a sustained-release theophylline formulation. Patients with severe exacerbation requiring systemic GC administration for ≥3 days or hospitalization more than once a year are also considered as asthmatics with GC-resistant disease.

5.4 Mechanism of Steroid Resistance

5.4.1 Genetic Background

Resistance to ICS treatment is an important indicator of severe asthma according to research on ICS responsiveness and genetic background [4, 5]. In genome-wide association studies, the gene encoding glucocorticoid-induced transcript 1 protein (GLCCl 1) has been identified as a factor for regulating ICS responsiveness. Patients with mutations in the gene for GLCC1L experienced less improvement in pulmonary function during ICS treatment. Future research is expected to further elucidate the association between ICS responsiveness and genetic background [5].

5.4.2 Functional Abnormalities of GRα and GRβ

In GC-resistant patients, a decrease in the binding capacity between GC and GRα has been observed in peripheral blood mononuclear cells (PBMC), e.g., T cells [6]. Interleukin (IL)-4 and IL-2 are elevated in bronchoalveolar lavage fluid (BALF) of GC-resistant patients, and stimulation of isolated PBMCs by IL-4 and IL-2 reproduces the decrease in the GC-GRα-binding capacity [7]. Moreover, when PBMCs collected from a GC-resistant asthma patient were cultured in a medium free from IL-4 and IL-2 for 48 hours, the binding capacity of GRα was restored, suggesting that the presence of IL-2 and IL-4 in the respiratory tract may affect the function of GRα. In GC-resistant asthma patients, impaired nuclear localization of GRα has been observed [8]. Recent reports indicate that protein phosphatase 2A (PP2A), which reverses phosphorylation of GRα, is related to the pathophysiology in patients with severe asthma [9, 10]. Thus, phosphorylated GRα might impair its nuclear import.

In addition, GRβ, the second splicing variant of the *GR* transcript, binds DNA but lacks affinity for GC and, therefore, antagonistically inhibits the action of GRα. Furthermore, enhanced expression of GRβ has been observed in inflammatory cells of the BALF fraction of GC-resistant asthma patients [11]. Previous reports indicated that GRβ decreased the activity of HDAC 2 [1, 12]. Hence, GRβ might be associated with GC resistance.

5.4.3 Transcription Factor Activation

It has been shown that expression of several transcription factors is elevated in patients with GC-resistant asthma. AP-1 is a dimeric transcription factor consisting of the subunits Jun and Fos, which is activated by c-Jun N-terminal kinases (JNK), a protein induced by inflammatory cytokines such as tumor necrosis factor (TNF)-α. Excessive AP-1 levels inhibit the binding of GRα to GRE. Importantly, AP-1 expression is elevated in patients with GC-resistant asthma, and previous reports indicated that the expression of JNK and AP-1 was difficult to suppress even after GC administration [13, 14].

5.4.4 Modification by Inflammatory Cells

A complex network of T2 cytokines, such as IL-4, IL-5, and IL-13, plays an important role in asthma pathology. These cytokines are produced by Th2, which are crucial for adaptive immunity. However, it has been recently reported that T2 cytokines are also produced by type 2 innate lymphoid cells (ILC2s), which mediate the innate immune response. Moreover, the neutrophilic inflammation induced by the Th17 cellular pathway also affects the pathogenesis of severe asthma. Th17 cells produce cytokines such as IL-17 and IL-22 that are involved in inducing neutrophilic inflammation. Modification of T-cell activity is also a contributing factor to GC resistance (Fig. 5.2).

5.4.4.1 Th17 Cells

Infiltration of neutrophils, along with eosinophils, occurs in the respiratory tract of severe asthma patients. However, ICS responsiveness decreases when the sputum neutrophil abundance exceeds 65% and the neutrophilic airway inflammation is presumed to cause GC resistance [15]. Immunocompetent Th17 cells express IL-17A, IL-17E, IL17-F, and IL-22 that induce neutrophilic airway inflammation by

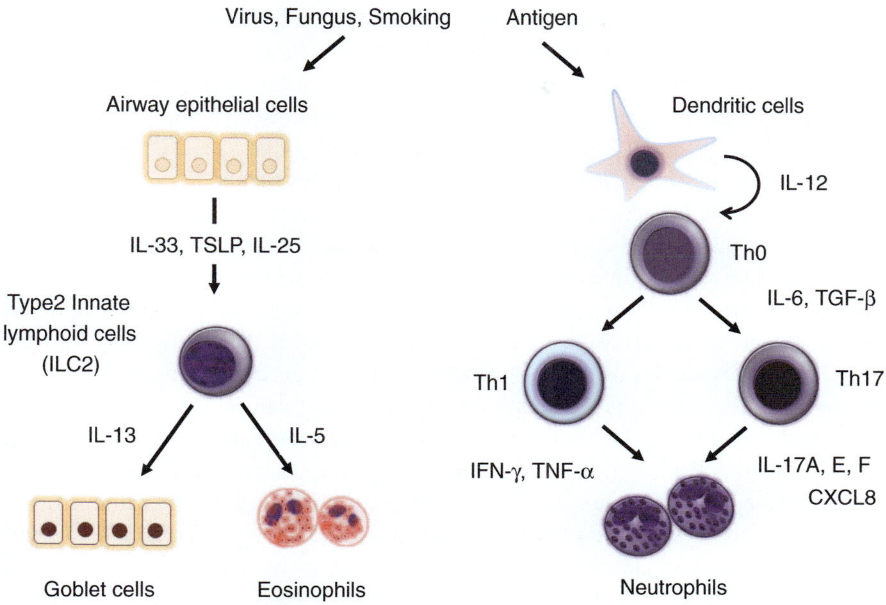

Fig. 5.2 Type 2 innate lymphoid cells and Th17 cells in asthma

stimulating the production of IL-8. In fact, the expression levels of IL-17A and IL17-F in the respiratory tract are correlated with neutrophilic inflammation and associated with asthma severity and GC resistance [16]. Moreover, recent reports indicated that IL-17A and IL-17F induced the expression of GRβ in respiratory epithelial cells, antagonizing the anti-inflammatory effect of GRα and facilitating the resistance to GC [17]. IL-8, which contributes to the activation of neutrophils and their accumulation in inflammation sites, is induced by lipopolysaccharide (LPS). Higher LPS levels are found in the BALF of GC-resistant asthma patients than in GC-responsive patients [18]. The LPS levels correlate with the expression of IL-8 mRNA derived from BALF cells in GC-resistant asthmatics [19]. Dysbiosis is common among asthmatic patients, associated with colonization pathogenic bacteria such as *Moraxella catarrhalis*, *Streptococcus pneumoniae*, or *Haemophilus influenzae*. Furthermore, in a study of BALF recovered from neutrophilic asthma patients, bacterial colonization was found in 55% of subjects [20]. It is conceivable that this type of bacterial colonization causes a shift in the pathology involving Th17 and Th1 cytokines that could induce GC resistance.

5.4.4.2 ILC2 Cells

It has been shown that T2 responses, typically required for adaptive immunity, do not necessarily occur in Th2 cells in asthmatic conditions. Immune response-induced pathogen-associated molecular patterns (PAMPs) released by microorganisms and damage-associated molecular patterns (DAMPs) released during autoimmune responses are initiated by innate immune cells. Natural killer (NK) cells are lymphocyte-like cells that are known to generate innate immunity. However, natural lymphocytes, ILC2 cells showing the same cytokine secretion as CD4+ T cells, have recently been identified. ILC2 do not possess T-cell or B-cell receptors. They are directly stimulated by cytokines such as IL-25 and IL-33 and thymic stromal lymphopoietin (TSLP), but not by an antigen-specific induction. ILC2 cells release T2 cytokines such as IL-5 and IL-13.

ILC2 cells in humans have been identified as lineage marker-negative, CD 127-positive, and CRTH 2-positive. They are found in various tissues and fluids such as the blood, lung, intestinal tract, as well as in nasal polyposis combined with chronic sinusitis. It has been recently reported that the ILC2 cell content is higher in the blood and alveolar lavage fluid of asthmatic patients than in healthy subjects [21, 22]. Interestingly, eosinophilic airway inflammation induced by IL-33 is suppressed by GC, whereas eosinophilic airway inflammation induced by IL-33 combined with TSLP is GC-resistant. Previous reports indicated that TSLP induced GC resistance in ILC2 cells by causing the phosphorylation of the signal transducer and activator of transcription 5 (STAT5) and upregulating the expression of anti-apoptotic B-cell lymphoma-extralarge (Bcl-xL) protein (Fig. 5.3) [23]. IL-33 and TSLP are induced in patients not only by severe asthma but also by virus infection, fungi, and proteases, which may contribute to the disease in patients with severe asthma. Importantly, a current report indicated that ILC2 cells isolated from asthma patients are more GC-resistant than Th2 cells [24]. Similarly, in a study comparing severe asthmatics with mild asthmatics, there was no difference in the number of Th2 cells, whereas the number of ILC 2 cells was higher in severe asthmatics than in mild asthmatics. Thus, the association of ILC2 cells with severe asthma and GC resistance suggests that these cells contribute to the pathology of the disease.

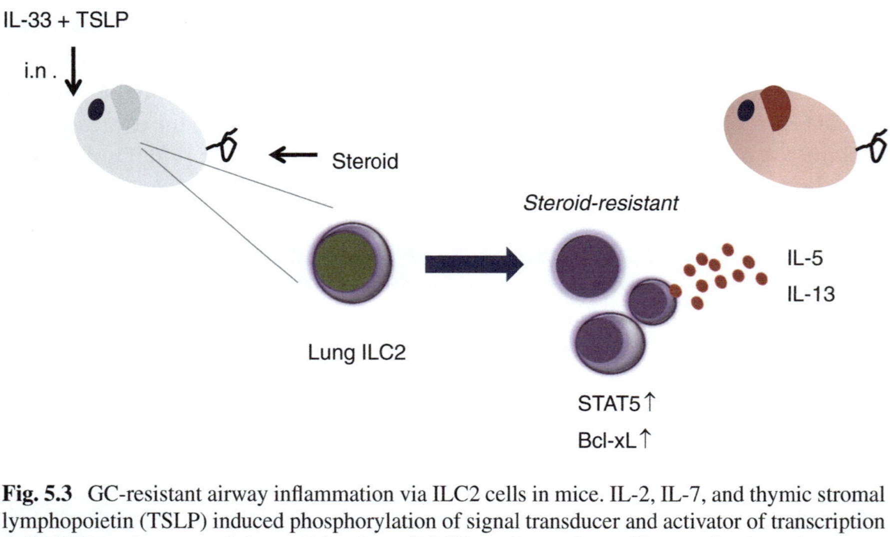

Fig. 5.3 GC-resistant airway inflammation via ILC2 cells in mice. IL-2, IL-7, and thymic stromal lymphopoietin (TSLP) induced phosphorylation of signal transducer and activator of transcription 5 (STAT5) and promoted the proliferation of ILC2s and type 2 cytokine production when combined with IL-33. TSLP, along with IL-33, induced phosphorylation of STAT5, promoted the proliferation of ILC2 cells, and induced type 2 cytokine production. TSLP also enhanced the expression of Bcl-xL, an anti-apoptotic factor

5.5 Clinical Phenotype

5.5.1 Obesity

Obesity is a typical phenotype of severe asthma that can cause systemic inflammation. In addition, excessive fatty acid content induces oxidative stress. Systemic inflammation is induced by upregulation of TLR2 and TLR4 expression and elevated NF-κB activity, causing an increase in TNF-α, IL-6, and C-reactive protein (CRP). Specifically, female obesity is associated with an increase in neutrophils in sputum, indicating a tendency to GC resistance [25, 26]. A recent study with obese, asthmatic mice, fed with a high-fat diet, indicated a crucial role for IL17A-producing ILC3 cells, and the NLRP3 inflammasome in disease progression IL1β was produced by macrophages, and ILC 3 cell numbers were increased in the lungs [27]. In addition, the increase in ILC3 cells correlated with the degree of airway hyperresponsiveness [21]. The number of ILC3 and airway hypersensitivity could be decreased by IL1 receptor antagonist.

5.5.2 Infection-Associated Asthma

Infection is one of the important asthma-exacerbating factors. Viral infections account for about 50% of the cases of exacerbation of adult asthma [28]. Influenza A, rhinovirus, and RSV infections frequently occur, and the effect of steroid therapy is reduced by viral infection [29–31]. Chlamydia respiratory tract infection may also contribute to GC resistance [32, 33]. Furthermore, it is reported that asthmatic patients who have potentially *Haemophilus influenzae* infection have non-eosinophilic asthma, requiring high doses of ICS [34]. Many infectious diseases cause neutrophilic inflammation by type 1 and type 17. Furthermore, it is shown in vivo that airway inflammation caused by allergens after infection causes GC resistance [35, 36]. Interestingly, response to TLR2, TLR4, IL-6, IL-1b, and NLRP3 as well as neutrophilic inflammation by type 1 or type 17 might be involved in exacerbation of asthma after infection, which contributes to GC resistance [37, 38].

5.6 Conclusion

Due to the widespread use of ICS, the disease can be controlled. However, ICS resistance is still reported in asthma patients. To elucidate the mechanism of GC resistance, we must consider the genetic background and various cell-related factors in association with asthma. Moreover, asthma is now studied as a disease that is linked to other syndromes responsible for comorbidities. Hence, the GC resistance might be linked to those comorbidity-causing syndromes. Future biomedical research needs to focus on this aspect.

References

1. Barnes PJ. Corticosteroid resistance in patients with asthma and chronic obstructive pulmonary disease. J Allergy Clin Immunol. 2013;131(3):636–45.
2. Adcock IM, Ford PA, Bhavsar P, Ahmad T, Chung KF. Steroid resistance in asthma: mechanisms and treatment options. Curr Allergy Asthma Rep. 2008;8(2):171–8.
3. Chung KF, Wenzel SE, Brozek JL, Bush A, Castro M, Sterk PJ, et al. International ERS/ATS guidelines on definition, evaluation and treatment of severe asthma. Eur Respir J. 2014;43(2):343–73.
4. ten Brinke A, Zwinderman AH, Sterk PJ, Rabe KF, Bel EH. "Refractory" eosinophilic airway inflammation in severe asthma: effect of parenteral corticosteroids. Am J Respir Crit Care Med. 2004;170(6):601–5.
5. Tantisira KG, Lasky-Su J, Harada M, Murphy A, Litonjua AA, Himes BE, et al. Genomewide association between GLCCI1 and response to glucocorticoid therapy in asthma. N Engl J Med. 2011;365(13):1173–83.
6. Sher ER, Leung DY, Surs W, Kam JC, Zieg G, Kamada AK, et al. Steroid-resistant asthma. Cellular mechanisms contributing to inadequate response to glucocorticoid therapy. J Clin Invest. 1994;93(1):33–9.
7. Leung DY, Martin RJ, Szefler SJ, Sher ER, Ying S, Kay AB, et al. Dysregulation of interleukin 4, interleukin 5, and interferon gamma gene expression in steroid-resistant asthma. J Exp Med. 1995;181(1):33–40.
8. Matthews JG, Ito K, Barnes PJ, Adcock IM. Defective glucocorticoid receptor nuclear translocation and altered histone acetylation patterns in glucocorticoid-resistant patients. J Allergy Clin Immunol. 2004;113(6):1100–8.
9. Kobayashi Y, Mercado N, Barnes PJ, Ito K. Defects of protein phosphatase 2A causes corticosteroid insensitivity in severe asthma. PLoS One. 2011;6(12):e27627.
10. Li JJ, Tay HL, Maltby S, Xiang Y, Eyers F, Hatchwell L, et al. MicroRNA-9 regulates steroid-resistant airway hyperresponsiveness by reducing protein phosphatase 2A activity. J Allergy Clin Immunol. 2015;136(2):462–73.
11. Goleva E, Li LB, Eves PT, Strand MJ, Martin RJ, Leung DY. Increased glucocorticoid receptor beta alters steroid response in glucocorticoid-insensitive asthma. Am J Respir Crit Care Med. 2006;173(6):607–16.
12. Li LB, Leung DY, Martin RJ, Goleva E. Inhibition of histone deacetylase 2 expression by elevated glucocorticoid receptor beta in steroid-resistant asthma. Am J Respir Crit Care Med. 2010;182(7):877–83.
13. Loke TK, Mallett KH, Ratoff J, O'Connor BJ, Ying S, Meng Q, et al. Systemic glucocorticoid reduces bronchial mucosal activation of activator protein 1 components in glucocorticoid-sensitive but not glucocorticoid-resistant asthmatic patients. J Allergy Clin Immunol. 2006;118(2):368–75.
14. Hew M, Bhavsar P, Torrego A, Meah S, Khorasani N, Barnes PJ, et al. Relative corticosteroid insensitivity of peripheral blood mononuclear cells in severe asthma. Am J Respir Crit Care Med. 2006;174(2):134–41.
15. McWilliams T, Wells AU, Harrison AC, Lindstrom S, Cameron RJ, Foskin E. Induced sputum and bronchoscopy in the diagnosis of pulmonary tuberculosis. Thorax. 2002;57(12):1010–4.
16. Al-Ramli W, Prefontaine D, Chouiali F, Martin JG, Olivenstein R, Lemiere C, et al. T(H)17-associated cytokines (IL-17A and IL-17F) in severe asthma. J Allergy Clin Immunol. 2009;123(5):1185–7.
17. Vazquez-Tello A, Semlali A, Chakir J, Martin JG, Leung DY, Eidelman DH, et al. Induction of glucocorticoid receptor-beta expression in epithelial cells of asthmatic airways by T-helper type 17 cytokines. Clin Exp Allergy. 2010;40(9):1312–22.
18. Goleva E, Hauk PJ, Hall CF, Liu AH, Riches DW, Martin RJ, et al. Corticosteroid-resistant asthma is associated with classical antimicrobial activation of airway macrophages. J Allergy Clin Immunol. 2008;122(3):550.e3–9.e3.

19. McSharry C, Spears M, Chaudhuri R, Cameron EJ, Husi H, Thomson NC. Increased sputum endotoxin levels are associated with an impaired lung function response to oral steroids in asthmatic patients. J Allergy Clin Immunol. 2014;134(5):1068–75.
20. Liu W, Liu S, Verma M, Zafar I, Good JT, Rollins D, et al. Mechanism of TH2/TH17-predominant and neutrophilic TH2/TH17-low subtypes of asthma. J Allergy Clin Immunol. 2017;139(5):1548.e4–58.e4.
21. Morita H, Moro K, Koyasu S. Innate lymphoid cells in allergic and nonallergic inflammation. J Allergy Clin Immunol. 2016;138(5):1253–64.
22. Tojima I, Kouzaki H, Shimizu S, Ogawa T, Arikata M, Kita H, et al. Group 2 innate lymphoid cells are increased in nasal polyps in patients with eosinophilic chronic rhinosinusitis. Clin Immunol. 2016;170:1–8.
23. Kabata H, Moro K, Fukunaga K, Suzuki Y, Miyata J, Masaki K, et al. Thymic stromal lymphopoietin induces corticosteroid resistance in natural helper cells during airway inflammation. Nat Commun. 2013;4:2675.
24. Liu S, Verma M, Michalec L, Liu W, Sripada A, Rollins D, et al. Steroid resistance of airway type 2 innate lymphoid cells from patients with severe asthma: The role of thymic stromal lymphopoietin. J Allergy Clin Immunol. 2018;141(1):257.e6–68.e6.
25. Simpson JL, Scott R, Boyle MJ, Gibson PG. Inflammatory subtypes in asthma: assessment and identification using induced sputum. Respirology. 2006;11(1):54–61.
26. Scott HA, Gibson PG, Garg ML, Upham JW, Wood LG. Sex hormones and systemic inflammation are modulators of the obese-asthma phenotype. Allergy. 2016;71(7):1037–47.
27. Kim HY, Lee HJ, Chang YJ, Pichavant M, Shore SA, Fitzgerald KA, et al. Interleukin-17-producing innate lymphoid cells and the NLRP3 inflammasome facilitate obesity-associated airway hyperreactivity. Nat Med. 2014;20(1):54–61.
28. Atmar RL, Guy E, Guntupalli KK, Zimmerman JL, Bandi VD, Baxter BD, et al. Respiratory tract viral infections in inner-city asthmatic adults. Arch Intern Med. 1998;158(22):2453–9.
29. Hansbro NG, Horvat JC, Wark PA, Hansbro PM. Understanding the mechanisms of viral induced asthma: new therapeutic directions. Pharmacol Ther. 2008;117(3):313–53.
30. Gerke AK, Yang M, Tang F, Foster ED, Cavanaugh JE, Polgreen PM. Association of hospitalizations for asthma with seasonal and pandemic influenza. Respirology. 2014;19(1):116–21.
31. Wark PA, Johnston SL, Moric I, Simpson JL, Hensley MJ, Gibson PG. Neutrophil degranulation and cell lysis is associated with clinical severity in virus-induced asthma. Eur Respir J. 2002;19(1):68–75.
32. Patel KK, Vicencio AG, Du Z, Tsirilakis K, Salva PS, Webley WC. Infectious Chlamydia pneumoniae is associated with elevated interleukin-8 and airway neutrophilia in children with refractory asthma. Pediatr Infect Dis J. 2010;29(12):1093–8.
33. Black PN, Scicchitano R, Jenkins CR, Blasi F, Allegra L, Wlodarczyk J, et al. Serological evidence of infection with Chlamydia pneumoniae is related to the severity of asthma. Eur Respir J. 2000;15(2):254–9.
34. Green BJ, Wiriyachaiporn S, Grainge C, Rogers GB, Kehagia V, Lau L, et al. Potentially pathogenic airway bacteria and neutrophilic inflammation in treatment resistant severe asthma. PLoS One. 2014;9(6):e100645.
35. Essilfie AT, Horvat JC, Kim RY, Mayall JR, Pinkerton JW, Beckett EL, et al. Macrolide therapy suppresses key features of experimental steroid-sensitive and steroid-insensitive asthma. Thorax. 2015;70(5):458–67.
36. Kim RY, Horvat JC, Pinkerton JW, Starkey MR, Essilfie AT, Mayall JR, et al. MicroRNA-21 drives severe, steroid-insensitive experimental asthma by amplifying phosphoinositide 3-kinase-mediated suppression of histone deacetylase 2. J Allergy Clin Immunol. 2017;139(2):519–32.
37. Kim RY, Pinkerton JW, Essilfie AT, Robertson AAB, Baines KJ, Brown AC, et al. Role for NLRP3 inflammasome-mediated, IL-1beta-dependent responses in severe, steroid-resistant asthma. Am J Respir Crit Care Med. 2017;196(3):283–97.
38. Essilfie AT, Simpson JL, Dunkley ML, Morgan LC, Oliver BG, Gibson PG, et al. Combined Haemophilus influenzae respiratory infection and allergic airways disease drives chronic infection and features of neutrophilic asthma. Thorax. 2012;67(7):588–99.

Part II
Diagnosis

Chapter 6
Asthma Phenotype and Endotype

Satoshi Konno

Abstract Asthma has been recognized as a heterogeneous and genetically complex disease that cannot be explained with a single mechanism. Asthma comprises a number of disease variants with different underlying pathophysiologies. Recently, the term "precision medicine" has been proposed and defined as "treatments targeted to the needs of individual patients on the basis of genetic, biomarker, phenotypic, or psychosocial characteristics that distinguish a given patient from other patients with similar clinical presentations." In the context of chronic airways diseases, precision medicine can therefore be a promising strategy to improve management. Precision medicine is based on integrated assessment of the complex clinical and biological status of individual patients, based on the concept of "phenotype," "endotype," and "treatable traits." This section summarizes the recent concept of these terms toward the accomplishment of treating asthmatic subjects.

Keywords Phenotype · Endotype · Cluster analysis · Diagnosis · Treatable traits

6.1 What Is Phenotype/Endotype?

A number of molecules have been proposed as novel therapeutic targets in the treatment of asthma, based on results in murine models [1]. However, few new treatments for human asthma have been developed since the introduction of inhaled corticosteroids, though several clinical trials with this aim have been conducted. The main reason for these disappointing results is our limited knowledge of the

S. Konno (✉)
Department of Respiratory Medicine, Faculty of Medicine and Graduate School of Medicine, Hokkaido University, Sapporo, Hokkaido, Japan
e-mail: satkonno@med.hokudai.ac.jp

A. Yokoyama (ed.), *Advances in Asthma*, Respiratory Disease Series: Diagnostic Tools and Disease Managements, https://doi.org/10.1007/978-981-13-2790-2_6

Table 6.1 Potential phenotypic classifications in asthmatic subjects

Child onset	Adult onset
High IgE	Low IgE
Atopic	Nonatopic
Eosinophilic	Non-eosinophilic
High FeNO	Low FeNO
Smoking	Non-smoking
Obese	Nonobese
With sinusitis	Without sinusitis
AERD	Non-AERD
Frequent exacerbation	Non-exacerbation

pathogenesis of human asthma. Recently, human asthma has been recognized as a heterogeneous and genetically complex disease that cannot be explained with a single mechanism. Asthma comprises a number of disease variants with different underlying pathophysiologies. In recent years, the concept of "phenotype" has become increasingly important in the study of asthma.

A phenotype (from Greek *phainein*, meaning "to show," and *typos*, meaning "type") is the composite of an organism's observable characteristics or traits, such as morphology, development, biochemical or physiological properties, behavior, and products of behavior [2]. A phenotype results from the expression of an organism's genetic code, its genotype, as well as the influence of environmental factors and the interactions between the two. Table 6.1 shows representative phenotypes of asthma, which could be applicable in current clinical practice. The concept of phenotype suggests that distinct therapeutic approaches depending on different phenotypes would be necessary.

In contrast with phenotype, an "endotype" is a subtype of a condition, defined based on a distinct functional or pathobiological mechanism [3, 4]. This is distinct from phenotype, which is any observable characteristic or trait of a disease, such as morphology, development, biochemical or physiological properties, or behavior, without any implication of a mechanism. It is envisaged that patients with a specific endotype present themselves within phenotypic clusters of diseases. In other words, endotype is used to describe a subtype of a disease defined based on a unique or distinctive functional or pathophysiological mechanism. A more extensive rational approach is to assess components of asthma that may be considered per the definition of endotypes. The asthma endotype model has shown associations between clinical determinants that are known to be important in the manifestation and expression of asthma across its diverse patterns and severities.

6.2 Cluster Analysis

Cluster analysis is the task of grouping a set of objects in such a way that objects in the same group are more similar to each other than to those in other groups. It is a primary task in exploratory data mining, and a common technique in statistical data

Table 6.2 Representative reports using cluster analysis in asthmatic subjects

Author	Study name	Population	Journal	Year
Haldar P, et al.	Leicester study	Asthma	AJRCCM	2008
Moore WC, et al.	SARP	Asthma	AJRCCM	2010
Moore WC, et al.	SARP	Asthma	JACI	2013
Wu W, et al.	SARP	Asthma + HV	JACI	2014
Schatz M, et al.	TENOR	Difficult-to-treat asthma	JACI	2013
Amelink M		Adult-onset asthma	Allergy	2013
Kim TB, et al.	COREA	Asthma	Eur Respir J	2013
Jang AS, et al.	COREA	Severe asthma	Lung	2013
Kaneko Y, et al.		Asthma	Allergol Int	2013
Nagasaki T, et al.	KiHAC	Asthma	JACI	2014
Konno, et al.	HiCARAT	Severe asthma	Ann Am Thorac Soc	2018
Tanaka, et al.	IAI	Asthma exacerbation	Allergy	2018

analysis used in several fields including machine learning, pattern recognition, image analysis, information retrieval, bioinformatics, data compression, and computer graphics. This classification approach has recently been also applied to explore and characterize novel asthma phenotypes, which are not based on any a priori hypotheses. Table 6.2 shows representative reports using this approach in asthmatic subjects [5–13].

However, it should be borne in mind that cluster analysis has some inherent limitations, including the somewhat intentional variable selection, with potential biases toward researchers' interests [5–7]. Although variables have been selected statistically in some studies in an attempt to reduce their redundancy and to enhance stability of the analysis [8–11], the results would be highly affected by the variables selected. We should therefore consider this analysis as a process of knowledge discovery via classification of subjects into a limited number of clusters on the basis of our existing knowledge and an a priori hypothesis. This is a significant step toward a stronger hypothesis beginning with a premature hypothesis.

6.3 Limitation of Classification of Subjects Based on Phenotypes/Endotypes

As mentioned above, phenotyping or endotyping would certainly be a useful way to classify heterogenous diseases such as asthma and COPD. However, it is important to consider that classifications of subjects into two or three groups per phenotypes/endotypes are based on the concept that the effect of any single factor the disease is has the same directional trend in all subjects. For example, smoking and obesity have multifactorial effects on asthma phenotypes, although they are generally considered to have deleterious effects on asthma [14]. For clarification, investigators have classified the disease into groups such as smokers and nonsmokers, or obese and nonobese, and compared asthma phenotypes between the groups. However, reports have been highly inconsistent, especially with regard to the effects of smoking on airway inflammation in asthma; some studies have demonstrated that smoking attenuates eosinophilic inflammation, whereas others report eosinophilic inflammation induced by smoking in human and animal studies. Thus, if we hypothesize that the effect of several factors (i.e., smoking, obesity) does not have the same directional trend, the strategy for classification of subjects into groups would not clarify their effects on asthma phenotypes in individual subjects.

In our recent report in particular, we hypothesized that the effects of smoking on inflammation in asthma would vary and would not affect all subjects similarly. It was anticipated that cluster analysis would clarify this complexity. We conducted cluster analysis, and it provided two distinct phenotypes with potentially different biological pathways contributing to fixed airflow limitation in cigarette smokers with severe asthma [12]. We surmise that these results should facilitate further studies to confirm the differential effects of smoking on airway inflammation in individuals.

6.4 What Does "Diagnosis" Mean?

Recently, the term "precision medicine" has been proposed and defined as "treatments targeted to the needs of individual patients on the basis of genetic, biomarker, phenotypic, or psychosocial characteristics that distinguish a given patient from other patients with similar clinical presentations" [15]. In the context of chronic airways diseases, precision medicine can therefore be a promising strategy to improve management. Needless to say, physicians always try to be as precise as possible in relation to the needs of individual patients. The above change toward precision medicine, however, is based on integrated assessment of the complex clinical and biological status of individual patients, which until recently was beyond reach.

Dr. Shigeaki Hinohara has stated that "diagnosis" is composed of two words, "dia" and "gnosis"; "dia" means "to know," and "gnosis" means "thoroughly." He emphasized that diagnosis is not the way to name a disease but to consider the best method of treatment based on the patient's condition and tests. Naming the disease may not the matter for patients, but rather, selection of the best treatments regardless of the name of the disease is crucial.

The term "treatable trait" is a therapeutic target identified based on "phenotype" or "endotype" recognition through validated biomarker(s) [16]. Table 6.3 lists a number of potential pulmonary, extrapulmonary, and behavioral/lifestyle treatable traits to consider in patients with asthma and their specific therapeutic recommendations per current international recommendations. These concepts are not captured adequately by the traditional phenotype concept and are therefore important for the clinician to understand. Finally, we would also like to emphasize that the concept of "finding the treatable traits" could be applied not only to asthma but also to other

Table 6.3 Examples of treatable traits of asthma

Treatable traits	Diagnostic criteria	Treatment
Smoking habit		Smoking cessation
Obesity		Education
Exposure to agents/pollutions		Avoidance
Airway inflammation	Blood test, FeNO, sputum	
	Eosinophilic	Corticosteroid
	Neutrophilic	Macrolides
Airflow limitation	Spirometry	Bronchodilators
Hypoxemia	Blood gas analysis, SpO_2	Oxygen therapy
		Noninvasive ventilation
Chronic bronchitis	Sputum	Carbocysteine macrolides
Airway bacterial colonization	Sputum	Macrolides
Precapillary pulmonary hypertension	Echocardiography Right heart catheterization	Vasodilators
Adherence		Education
Comorbidities		

refractory pulmonary diseases such as COPD, interstitial pneumonia, ARDS, and pulmonary hypertension.

References

1. Adcock IM, Caramori G, Chung KF. New targets for drug development in asthma. Lancet. 2008;20:1073–87.
2. Wikipedia. https://en.wikipedia.org/wiki/Phenotype.
3. Anderson GP. Endotyping asthma: new insights into key pathogenic mechanisms in a complex, heterogeneous disease. Lancet. 2008;20:1107–19.
4. Wikipedia. https://en.wikipedia.org/wiki/Endotype.
5. Haldar P, Pavord ID, Shaw DE, Berry MA, Thomas M, Brightling CE, Wardlaw AJ, Green RH. Cluster analysis and clinical asthma phenotypes. Am J Respir Crit Care Med. 2008;178:218–24.
6. Moore WC, Meyers DA, Wenzel SE, Teague WG, Li H, Li X, D'Agostino R Jr, Castro M, Curran-Everett D, Fitzpatrick AM, Gaston B, Jarjour NN, Sorkness R, Calhoun WJ, Chung KF, Comhair SA, Dweik RA, Israel E, Peters SP, Busse WW, Erzurum SC, Bleecker ER, National Heart, Lung, and Blood Institute's Severe Asthma Research Program. Identification of asthma phenotypes using cluster analysis in the Severe Asthma Research Program. Am J Respir Crit Care Med. 2010;181:315–23.
7. Kim TB, Jang AS, MD KHS, Park JS, Chang YS, Cho SH, Choi BW, Park JW, MD NDH, Yoon HJ, Cho YJ, Moon HB, Cho YS, Choon-Sik Park CS. Identification of asthma clusters in two independent Korean adult asthma cohorts. Eur Respir J. 2013;41:1308–14.
8. Amelink M, de Nijs SB, de Groot JC, van Tilburg PM, van Spiegel PI, Krouwels FH, Lutter R, Zwinderman AH, Weersink EJ, ten Brinke A, Sterk PJ, Bel EH. Three phenotypes of adult-onset asthma. Allergy. 2013;68:674–80.
9. Schatz M, Hsu JW, Zeiger RS, Chen W, Dorenbaum A, Chipps BE, Haselkorn T. Phenotypes determined by cluster analysis in severe or difficult-to-treat asthma. J Allergy Clin Immunol. 2014;133:1549–56.

10. Moore WC, Hastie AT, Li X, Li H, Busse WW, Jarjour NN, Wenzel SE, Peters SP, Meyers DA, Bleecker ER, National Heart, Lung, and Blood Institute's Severe Asthma Research Program. Sputum neutrophil counts are associated with more severe asthma phenotypes using cluster analysis. J Allergy Clin Immunol. 2014;133:1557–63.
11. Wu W, Bleecker E, Moore W, Busse WW, Castro M, Chung KF, Calhoun WJ, Erzurum S, Gaston B, Elliot Israel E, Curran-Everett D, Wenzel SE. Unsupervised phenotyping of severe asthma research program participants using expanded lung data. J Allergy Clin Immunol. 2014;133:1280–8.
12. Konno S, Taniguchi N, Makita H, Nakamaru Y, Shimizu K, Shijubo N, Fuke S, Takeyabu K, Oguri M, Kimura H, Maeda Y, Suzuki M, Nagai K, Ito YM, Wenzel SE, Nishimura M. Distinct phenotypes of smokers with fixed airflow limitation identified by cluster analysis of severe asthma. Ann Am Thorac Soc. 2018;15:33–41.
13. Tanaka H, Nakatani E, Fukutomi Y, Sekiya K, Kaneda H, Iikura M, Yoshida M, Takahashi K, Tomii K, Nishikawa M, Kaneko N, Sugino Y, Shinkai M, Ueda T, Tanikawa Y, Shirai T, Hirabayashi M, Aoki T, Kato T, Iizuka K, Fujii M, Taniguchi M. Identification of patterns of factors preceding severe or life-threatening asthma exacerbations in a nationwide study. Allergy. 2018;73(5):1110–8.
14. Polosa R, Thomson NC. Smoking and asthma: dangerous liaisons. Eur Respir J. 2013;41:716–26.
15. Collins FS, Varmus H. A new initiative on precision medicine. N Engl J Med. 2015;26:793–5.
16. Agusti A, Bel E, Thomas M, Vogelmeier C, Brusselle G, Holgate S, Humbert M, Jones P, Gibson PG, Vestbo J, Beasley R, Pavord ID. Treatable traits: toward precision medicine of chronic airway diseases. Eur Respir J. 2016;47:410–9.

Chapter 7
Periostin as a Biomarker for Type 2 Asthma

Kenji Izuhara, Satoshi Nunomura, Junya Ono, Masayuki Takai, and Yasuhiro Nanri

Abstract Periostin is a protein having two characteristics—an extracellular matrix (ECM) protein important for maintaining tissue or organ structures and in generating fibrosis by binding to other ECM proteins and a matricellular protein transducing intracellular signaling by binding to several integrins on the cell surface. IL-4 and IL-13, signature type 2 cytokines abundantly expressed in the inflamed sites of asthma, induce periostin in several tissue-resident cells—fibroblasts, airway epithelial cells, and endothelial cells—and then periostin contributes to generating thick basement membranes, a typical histological feature in asthma patients. Periostin would play a role in accelerating airway allergic inflammation in asthma by acting as a matricellular protein. Serum periostin has characteristics as a biomarker, reflecting both type 2 inflammation and remodeling/fibrosis in asthma patients. These characteristics are useful for stratifying asthma patients and can predict the ICS resistance or efficacy of molecularly targeted drugs such as IL-4/IL-13 antagonists for asthma patients.

Keywords Biomarker · Matricellular protein · Molecularly targeted drug · IL-4 · IL-13

K. Izuhara (✉) · S. Nunomura · Y. Nanri
Division of Medical Biochemistry, Department of Biomolecular Sciences, Saga Medical School, Saga-shi, Saga, Japan
e-mail: kizuhara@cc.saga-u.ac.jp

J. Ono · M. Takai
Division of Medical Biochemistry, Department of Biomolecular Sciences, Saga Medical School, Saga-shi, Saga, Japan

Shino-Test Corporation, Sagamihara-shi, Kanagawa, Japan

A. Yokoyama (ed.), *Advances in Asthma*, Respiratory Disease Series: Diagnostic Tools and Disease Managements, https://doi.org/10.1007/978-981-13-2790-2_7

7.1 Introduction

Periostin was originally identified in 1993 as osteoblast-specific factor 2, a molecule highly expressed in the mouse osteoblastic cell line MC3T3-E1 [1]. It was then renamed periostin in 1999 because it is preferentially expressed in the periosteum and in periodontal ligaments [2].

Periostin has two characteristics: an extracellular matrix (ECM) protein and a matricellular protein [3, 4]. Periostin has a cysteine-rich EMILIN (EMI) domain at the N terminus and four fasciclin (FAS) 1 domains in the middle. These domains are important for binding to other ECM proteins such as collagen 1, fibronectin (EMI domain), and tenascin-C (FAS1 domain). Such functions of periostin as an ECM protein are important for maintaining tissue or organ structures in physiological conditions and in generating fibrosis in pathological conditions. Additionally, periostin binds to several integrins on the cell surface, transducing intracellular signaling via FAK, PI3-kinase, Akt, ERK, NF-κB, STAT3, and so on [3]. That is why periostin is classified as a matricellular protein defined as an ECM protein binding to its receptor on cell surfaces and functioning in cell activation rather than in maintenance of tissue structure. The aspect of periostin as a matricellular protein is important in the onset of inflammatory conditions, including asthma. It has been shown that periostin is expressed in various pathological conditions or diseases—allergic diseases, pulmonary fibrosis, scleroderma, renal diseases, ocular diseases, and malignancies—and plays a role in accelerating those by acting as both an ECM protein and a matricellular protein [4–9].

In this chapter, we focus on the expression and functions of periostin in asthma and then explain the usefulness of periostin as a biomarker for asthma.

7.2 Expression of Periostin in Asthma

It is known that various triggers—TGF-β, angiotensin II, connective tissue growth factor 2, bone morphogenetic protein 2, mechanical stress, and stimuli from malignancies—induce periostin expression [10–12] (Fig. 7.1). We found for the first time that IL-4 and IL-13, signature type 2 cytokines, induce periostin [13, 14]. In our hands, both airway epithelial cells and lung fibroblasts express periostin at the mRNA level; lung fibroblasts, but not airway epithelial cells, secrete periostin protein following stimulation by IL-4 or IL-13. That is why periostin can be used as a surrogate biomarker for IL-4 or IL-13, as we will mention below. It was then reported that periostin is secreted from the basal side, but not from the apical side of airway epithelial cells stimulated by IL-13, using an air/liquid interface method in which one side of the airway epithelial cells faces air, whereas the other side faces liquid medium [15]. Moreover, it was reported that microvascular endothelial cells can secrete periostin by stimulation of IL-4 or IL-13 [16]. Thus, at least three kinds

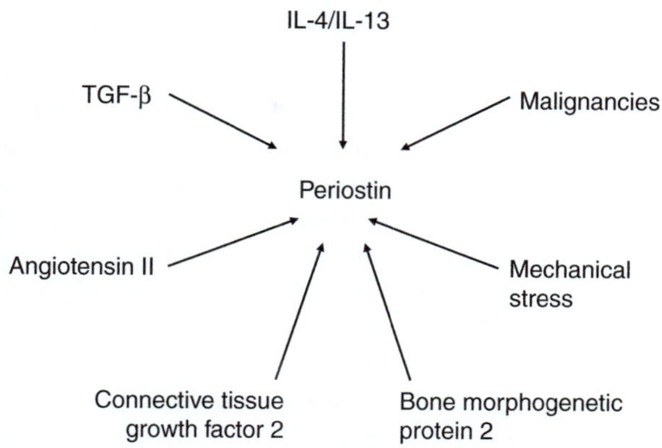

Fig. 7.1 Induction of periostin. Various triggers—IL-4/IL-13, TGF-β, angiotensin II, connective tissue growth factor 2, bone morphogenetic protein 2, mechanical stress, and stimuli from malignancies—induce periostin expression

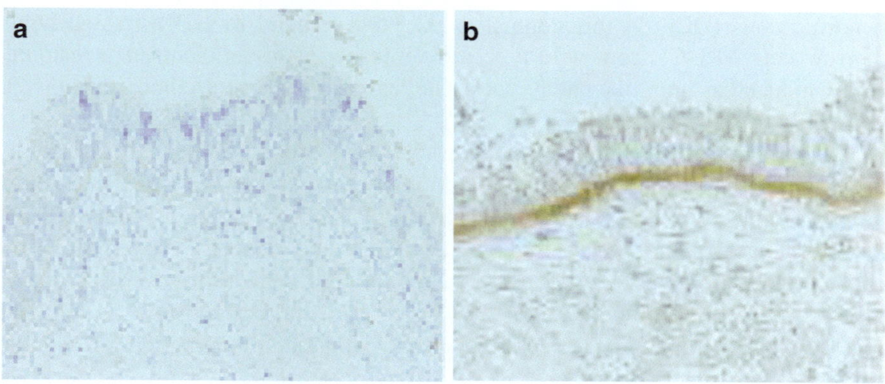

Fig. 7.2 High expression of periostin in asthma patients [14]. Periostin expression in bronchial tissues from a normal subject (**a**) and an asthma patient (**b**)

of tissue-resident cells in the lung—fibroblasts, epithelial cells, and endothelial cells—can produce periostin in response to IL-4 or IL-13.

Under normal conditions, periostin is only very weakly deposited in part of the bronchiolar basement membrane [17]. In contrast, periostin is robustly deposited on the thickened basement membrane in asthma patients, consistent with the notion that IL-4 and IL-13, triggers to induce periostin, are abundantly expressed in the bronchial tissues of these patients [14] (Fig. 7.2). Periostin is co-localized with collagens I, III, and V, fibronectin, and tenascin-C—all of them are ECM components of thickened basement membrane in asthma. This suggests that by binding to these ECM proteins, periostin thickens the basement membrane, a typical histological feature of asthma. In asthma patients, periostin in inflamed sites is likely to move easily to blood [18–20] and sputum [21, 22], although the precise mechanism of the movement or secretion remains elusive. That is also why periostin has an advantage as a biomarker for asthma.

7.3 Functions of Periostin in Asthma

Several trials to clarify the significance of periostin in the pathogenesis of asthma have been carried out using asthma model mice; however, the results are controversial and the conclusion remains uncertain. It was initially reported that when periostin-deficient mice were challenged with ovalbumin or *Aspergillus*, airway hyperresponsiveness (AHR), type 2 inflammation, and mucus production were also enhanced in these mice [23, 24]. These results suggested that periostin protects against allergic inflammation in these model mice. In contrast, Bentley et al. reported that all of these features—AHR, type 2 inflammation, and mucus production—were impaired in house dust mite (HDM)-challenged periostin-deficient mice and by administration of neutralizing anti-periostin antibodies [25]. These results suggested that, in contrast to the initial studies, periostin accelerates allergic inflammation in these model mice. They showed the importance of periostin in dendritic cells (DCs) in this context as adoptive transfer of HDM-treated bone marrow-derived DCs from wild-type mice into periostin-deficient mice restored HDM-induced asthma-like phenotypes. The reason for this contradiction is not yet known.

Kanemitsu *et al.* examined the importance of periostin deposition in asthma patients [26]. They analyzed the correlation between periostin expression in some biopsy samples that they took from asthma patients more than 20 years ago and recent changes of pulmonary function in those same patients. They found that deposition of periostin in the bronchial subepithelium in the samples was strongly inversely correlated with decline of ΔFEV1. These results support the notion that periostin plays a role in accelerating airway allergic inflammation in asthma patients.

We have examined the importance of periostin as a matricellular protein in the process of inflammation using *in vitro* systems. We have shown that particularly the involvement of periostin in the epithelial/mesenchymal interaction would be important for the pathogenesis of allergic diseases, including asthma (Fig. 7.3). In the three-dimensional organotypic co-culture system mimicking the epithelial/mesenchymal interaction in skin tissues, we showed that periostin derived from fibroblasts stimulated by IL-13 acts on keratinocytes by itself activating NF-κB inducing production of pro-inflammatory cytokines including TSLP [27]. Using the same system, we also showed that periostin acts on fibroblasts together with IL-1α activating NF-κB inducing IL-6 [28]. Moreover, we found that cooperative actions of periostin and either TNF-α or IL-1α activate NF-κB in lung fibroblasts, followed by production of MCP1/3, CXCL1/2, and IL-1β, pro-inflammatory cytokines important for recruiting neutrophils and macrophages [29]. These results point to the capability of periostin to activate NF-κB in tissue-resident cells such as epithelial cells and fibroblasts by itself or by cross talk with other pro-inflammatory mediators. Regarding periostin's actions on immune cells, it has been reported that it can act on eosinophils, inducing adhesion, superoxide generation, and TGF-β production [30, 31]. Thus, it is assumed that periostin plays various roles as a pro-inflammatory mediator acting on both tissue-resident cells and immune cells.

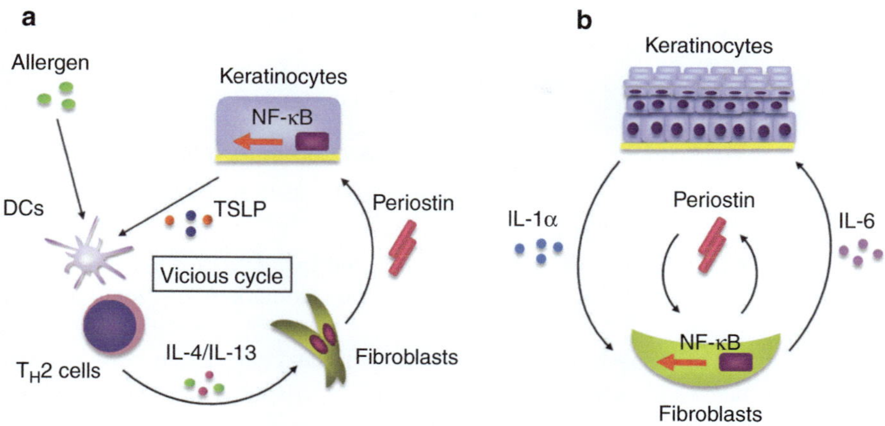

Fig. 7.3 Epithelial/mesenchymal interaction via periostin in the pathogenesis of allergic diseases [4]. (**a**) IL-4/IL-13 produced by T_H2 cells activated by exposure to allergens induces periostin production in fibroblasts. Periostin acts on keratinocytes, activating NF-κB followed by production of pro-inflammatory cytokines including TSLP, which acts on dendritic cells (DCs), accelerating type 2 inflammation. Thus, IL-4/IL-13, periostin, and TSLP generate a vicious cycle in the pathogenesis of skin allergic diseases. (**b**) IL-1α and periostin produced by keratinocytes and fibroblasts, respectively, cooperate to act on fibroblasts activating NF-κB. Activated fibroblasts produce IL-6 accelerating proliferation of keratinocytes

7.4 Periostin as a Biomarker for Asthma

7.4.1 A Biomarker for Type 2 (Th2-High) Asthma

It is now recognized that asthma is not a single disease but a syndrome [32]. We have empirically classified asthma patients based on clinical features such as age of onset (pediatric vs. adult), IgE dependency (atopic vs. nonatopic), and responsiveness to inhaled corticosteroids (ICSs, steroid-responsive vs. steroid-resistant). These classifications are based on phenotypes. In contrast, the significance of classifications based on molecular mechanisms of diseases, called endotypes, has recently emerged. Classifying asthma by type 2 vs. non-type 2 (or Th2-high vs. Th2-low) is an example of using endotypes [32]. This concept, "stratification of asthma patients," is the basis for applying molecularly targeted drugs for asthma, as we will discuss later.

The proportion of type 2 asthma defined by high expression of IL-5 and IL-13, signature type 2 cytokines, is estimated to be 50–70% of total asthma patients [33, 34]. Asano and his colleagues have recently estimated the proportion of type 2 in severe asthma patients to be ~80% in a Japanese population [35]. Fahy and his colleagues searched for biomarkers for type 2 asthma, finding that periostin is highly expressed in bronchial tissues of type 2 asthma patients together with chloride channel regulator 1 (CLCA1) and serpin peptidase inhibitor, clade B, member 2 (SERPINB2) [33]. They then found that serum periostin is high in type 2 asthma correlated with airway eosinophilia, compared to the fraction of exhaled nitric oxide

Fig. 7.4 Characteristics of periostin as a biomarker for asthma

- Reflection of type 2 inflammation and remodeling/fibrosis
- Resistance to ICSs
- Prediction of efficacy of molecularly targeted drugs for asthma, particularly IL-4/IL-13 antagonists

(FeNO), peripheral blood eosinophils, YKL-40, and IgE levels [34]. These results demonstrate that periostin has emerged as a novel biomarker for type 2 asthma (Fig. 7.4).

Our collaborators have intensively examined the characteristics of asthma patients correlated with serum periostin levels, using periostin ELISA kits with high sensitivity that we developed compared to other kits [36]. It has turned out that periostin is associated with eosinophil dominance [18–20, 37], late onset [18, 19], aspirin intolerance [19, 20], chronic sinusitis/olfactory dysfunction [18–20], and high FeNO [36–38]. These characteristics are known to be correlated with type 2 inflammation, which is consistent with the concept that periostin reflects type 2 inflammation. Moreover, these characteristics are known to be correlated with remodeling or fibrosis leading to resistance to treatments for asthma as we will mention next.

7.4.2 A Biomarker for ICS Resistance

We and our collaborators have shown that periostin is a component of the thickened basement membranes of asthma and is correlated with poor long-term prognosis [14, 26], suggesting that periostin has another characteristic as a biomarker for asthma reflecting remodeling or fibrosis. Matsumoto and her colleagues have demonstrated that periostin is associated with resistance to ICSs, the first-line drugs for asthma patients, which would be explained by this characteristic (Fig. 7.4). In the KiHAC study, when they divided asthma patients into rapid decliners and non-rapid decliners, defined by patients with treatments by ICS showing a decline in FEV_1 of more than or less than 30 mL/year, respectively, serum periostin was higher in rapid decliners than in non-rapid decliners. This suggests that serum periostin is associated with hyporesponsiveness to ICSs in asthma [18]. When they clustered these patients based on their peripheral eosinophil and neutrophil numbers, cluster 3, which was characterized by high eosinophils and low neutrophil numbers and late onset, showed that the difference in decline of FEV_1 between the periostin-high and periostin-low groups was more significant compared to the overall patients. This suggests that in this cluster, serum periostin is more associated with poor responsiveness to ICSs [39]. The association of serum periostin with poor responsiveness to ICSs was also observed in other studies [19, 36, 37]. Kato et al. showed more direct evidence for this association; when they tapered ICS treatment, asthma patients with high periostin showed a higher risk for instability than those with low periostin [40]. Introducing ICS to asthma patients promptly decreased FeNO levels, whereas it sustained high serum periostin levels. This finding suggests that ICS improves superficial inflammation consistent with decreased FeNO secreted from epithelial cells, whereas ICS does not improve the inflammation of deep layers consistent with sustained serum periostin [41]. Such limited efficacy of ICSs for asthma patients may lead to resistance to ICSs in periostin-high asthma patients showing high remodeling or fibrosis.

7.4.3 A Biomarker for Predicting the Efficacy of Molecularly Targeted Drugs for Type 2 Asthma

Currently, many drugs for type 2 asthma targeting IgE, IL-4/IL-13(receptor), IL-5(receptor), TSLP, CCR3, CCR4, CCL11, and CRTH2 are being developed. Some of them, two kinds of anti-IL-5 antibodies—mepolizumab and reslizumab—are already available at the start of 2018 [42]. Since periostin is a surrogate biomarker for type 2 asthma, particularly a downstream molecule of IL-4 and IL-13, several trials to apply periostin to a biomarker to predict efficacy of asthma drugs targeting IL-4 and IL-13 have been performed.

The first trial was carried out in the phase IIb study for lebrikizumab, an anti-IL-13 antibody, developed by Roche/Genentech [43]. They demonstrated that when they set the cutoff value of serum periostin at 50 ng/mL, the high periostin group showed good responsiveness to lebrikizumab, whereas the low periostin group showed poor responsiveness to it, demonstrating that serum periostin is a very useful biomarker to predict the efficacy of lebrikizumab. However, in the phase III study, lebrikizumab did not show enough efficacy for asthma patients, and development was ended [44]. In the phase IIb study of tralokinumab, another anti-IL-13 antibody, developed by AstraZeneca/MedImmune, both periostin and DPP-4, another type 2 biomarker, showed good ability to discriminate between good and poor responders to it as well as to lebrikizumab [45]. It is now in phase III study. Sanofi/Regeneron has developed dupilumab, an anti-IL-4 receptor α chain antibody that inhibits both IL-4 and IL-13 signals, as the first molecularly targeted drug for atopic dermatitis [46]. They have also developed dupilumab as an anti-asthma drug. In the phase IIb study, they used the blood eosinophil number as a biomarker to stratify patients; however, although the high eosinophil group tended to respond better than the low eosinophil group, dupilumab showed statistically significant efficacy in both groups [47]. It is also now in phase III.

We have examined the ability of serum periostin for this purpose instead of blood eosinophil number using the same samples as a post hoc study, finding that serum periostin showed a good ability to discriminate between good and poor responders as defined by improved lung functions (unpublished data, presented at the ERS Congress, 2016). Taken together, serum periostin has the potential to be a useful biomarker to predict the efficacy of IL-4/IL-13 antagonists (Fig. 7.4).

The usefulness of periostin as a biomarker to predict of efficacy of molecularly targeted drugs for type 2 asthma was examined for omalizumab, an anti-IgE antibody, provided by Novartis/Genentech. At this point, two studies have shown its usefulness [48, 49]. To our knowledge, these are the only studies so far to examine the usefulness of serum periostin as a biomarker to predict efficacy of molecularly targeted drugs for type 2 asthma except IL-4/IL-13 antagonists. These results point to the possibility that serum periostin is useful to predict efficacy of more molecularly targeted drugs for type 2 asthma other than IL-4/IL-13 antagonists.

7.5 Conclusion

It is strongly suggested that periostin acts as a pro-inflammatory mediator in asthma, although it has not been conclusively shown. Moreover, the usefulness of periostin as a biomarker for asthma—reflection of type 2 inflammation, resistance to ICS treatment, and prediction efficacy of several anti-asthma drugs targeting type 2 asthma—has been demonstrated. However, there still remain unresolved issues in this field—the pathological role of periostin in asthma, the usefulness of periostin as a biomarker to predict efficacy of molecularly targeted drugs for asthma, and the development of periostin detection systems more suitable for treating asthma patients. We need to begin to address these questions now.

Acknowledgments We thank Dr. Dovie R. Wylie for the critical review of this manuscript. We also thank the following colleagues and collaborators for contributing to the present work: Go Takayama, Masaru Uchida, Miho Masuoka, Hiroshi Shiraishi, Kanako Ontsuka, Kazuto Taniguchi, Yasutaka Mitamura, Tomohito Yoshihara, Kazuhiko Arima, Shoichi Suzuki, Shoichiro Ohta, Go Kato, Koichiro Takahashi, Shin-ichiro Hayashi (Saga Medical School), Noriko Yuyama (Genox Research, Inc.), Akihiro Ishida, Nobuo Ohta (Yamagata University), Hiroshi Fujishima (Tsurumi University), Naoko Okada, Kenji Matsumoto (National Research Institute for Child Health and Development Laboratory), Yoshihiro Kanemitsu, Tadao Nagasaki, Tomoko Tajiri, Hisako Matsumoto (Kyoto University), Masako Matsuzaka, Koichi Fukunaga (Keio University), Koichiro Asano (Tokai University), Yorihisa Kotobuki, Ichiro Katayama (Osaka University), Kenzen Kou, Yukie Yamaguchi, Michiko Aihara (Yokohama City University), Timothy Hinks, Peter Howarth (Southampton University Hospital), Mi-Ae Kim, Hae-Sim Park (Ajou University), Anna James, Sven-Erik Dahlen (Karolinska Institutet), Ayami Kamei, Yoshinori Azuma (Shino-Test Co.), Simon J. Conway (Indiana University), Masaki Okamoto, Tomoaki Hoshino, and Kiminori Fujimoto (Kurume University).

References

1. Takeshita S, Kikuno R, Tezuka K, Amann E. Osteoblast-specific factor 2: cloning of a putative bone adhesion protein with homology with the insect protein fasciclin I. Biochem J. 1993;294:271–8.
2. Horiuchi K, Amizuka N, Takeshita S, Takamatsu H, Katsuura M, Ozawa H, et al. Identification and characterization of a novel protein, periostin, with restricted expression to periosteum and

periodontal ligament and increased expression by transforming growth factor β. J Bone Miner Res. 1999;14:1239–49.
3. Izuhara K, Arima K, Ohta S, Suzuki S, Inamitsu M, Yamamoto K. Periostin in allergic inflammation. Allergol Int. 2014;63:143–51.
4. Izuhara K, Nunomura S, Nanri Y, Ogawa M, Ono J, Mitamura Y, et al. Periostin in inflammation and allergy. Cell Mol Life Sci. 2017;74:4293–303.
5. O'Dwyer DN, Moore BB. The role of periostin in lung fibrosis and airway remodeling. Cell Mol Life Sci. 2017;74:4305–14.
6. Murota H, Lingli Y, Katayama I. Periostin in the pathogenesis of skin diseases. Cell Mol Life Sci. 2017;74:4321–8.
7. Prakoura N, Chatziantoniou C. Periostin in kidney diseases. Cell Mol Life Sci. 2017;74: 4315–20.
8. Yoshida S, Nakama T, Ishikawa K, Nakao S, Sonoda KH, Ishibashi T. Periostin in vitreoretinal diseases. Cell Mol Life Sci. 2017;74:4329–37.
9. Cui D, Huang Z, Liu Y, Ouyang G. The multifaceted role of periostin in priming the tumor microenvironments for tumor progression. Cell Mol Life Sci. 2017;74:4287–91.
10. Conway SJ, Izuhara K, Kudo Y, Litvin J, Markwald R, Ouyang G, et al. The role of periostin in tissue remodeling across health and disease. Cell Mol Life Sci. 2014;71:1279–88.
11. Nishida M, Sato Y, Uemura A, Narita Y, Tozaki-Saitoh H, Nakaya M, et al. P2Y6 receptor-Gα12/13 signalling in cardiomyocytes triggers pressure overload-induced cardiac fibrosis. EMBO J. 2008;27:3104–15.
12. Liu AY, Zheng H, Ouyang G. Periostin, a multifunctional matricellular protein in inflammatory and tumor microenvironments. Matrix Biol. 2014;37:150–6.
13. Yuyama N, Davies DE, Akaiwa M, Matsui K, Hamasaki Y, Suminami Y, et al. Analysis of novel disease-related genes in bronchial asthma. Cytokine. 2002;19:287–96.
14. Takayama G, Arima K, Kanaji T, Toda S, Tanaka H, Shoji S, et al. Periostin: a novel component of subepithelial fibrosis of bronchial asthma downstream of IL-4 and IL-13 signals. J Allergy Clin Immunol. 2006;118:98–104.
15. Sidhu SS, Yuan S, Innes AL, Kerr S, Woodruff PG, Hou L, et al. Roles of epithelial cell-derived periostin in TGF-β activation, collagen production, and collagen gel elasticity in asthma. Proc Natl Acad Sci U S A. 2010;107:14170–5.
16. Shoda T, Futamura K, Kobayashi F, Saito H, Matsumoto K, Matsuda A. Cell type-dependent effects of corticosteroid on periostin production by primary human tissue cells. Allergy. 2013;68:1467–70.
17. Okamoto M, Hoshino T, Kitasato Y, Sakazaki Y, Kawayama T, Fujimoto K, et al. Periostin, a matrix protein, is a novel biomarker for idiopathic interstitial pneumonias. Eur Respir J. 2011;37:1119–27.
18. Kanemitsu Y, Matsumoto H, Izuhara K, Tohda Y, Kita H, Horiguchi T, et al. Increased periostin associates with greater airflow limitation in patients receiving inhaled corticosteroids. J Allergy Clin Immunol. 2013;132:305–12.
19. Matsusaka M, Kabata H, Fukunaga K, Suzuki Y, Masaki K, Mochimaru T, et al. Phenotype of asthma related with high serum periostin levels. Allergol Int. 2015;64:175–80.
20. Kim MA, Izuhara K, Ohta S, Ono J, Yoon MK, Ban GY, et al. Association of serum periostin with aspirin-exacerbated respiratory disease. Ann Allergy Asthma Immunol. 2014;113: 314–20.
21. Bobolea I, Barranco P, Del Pozo V, Romero D, Sanz V, Lopez-Carrasco V, et al. Sputum periostin in patients with different severe asthma phenotypes. Allergy. 2015;70:540–6.
22. Simpson JL, Yang IA, Upham JW, Reynolds PN, Hodge S, James AL, et al. Periostin levels and eosinophilic inflammation in poorly-controlled asthma. BMC Pulm Med. 2016;16:67.
23. Sehra S, Yao W, Nguyen ET, Ahyi AN, Tuana FM, Ahlfeld SK, et al. Periostin regulates goblet cell metaplasia in a model of allergic airway inflammation. J Immunol. 2011;186:4959–66.
24. Gordon ED, Sidhu SS, Wang ZE, Woodruff PG, Yuan S, Solon MC, et al. A protective role for periostin and TGF-β in IgE-mediated allergy and airway hyperresponsiveness. Clin Exp Allergy. 2012;42:144–55.

25. Bentley JK, Chen Q, Hong JY, Popova AP, Lei J, Moore BB, et al. Periostin is required for maximal airways inflammation and hyperresponsiveness in mice. J Allergy Clin Immunol. 2014;134:1433–42.
26. Kanemitsu Y, Ito I, Niimi A, Izuhara K, Ohta S, Ono J, et al. Osteopontin and periostin are associated with a 20-year decline of pulmonary function in patients with asthma. Am J Respir Crit Care Med. 2014;190:472–4.
27. Masuoka M, Shiraishi H, Ohta S, Suzuki S, Arima K, Aoki S, et al. Periostin promotes chronic allergic inflammation in response to Th2 cytokines. J Clin Invest. 2012;122:2590–600.
28. Taniguchi K, Arima K, Masuoka M, Ohta S, Shiraishi H, Ontsuka K, et al. Periostin controls keratinocyte proliferation and differentiation by interacting with the paracrine IL-1α/IL-6 loop. J Invest Dermatol. 2014;134:1295–304.
29. Uchida M, Shiraishi H, Ohta S, Arima K, Taniguchi K, Suzuki S, et al. Periostin, a matricellular protein, plays a role in the induction of chemokines in pulmonary fibrosis. Am J Respir Cell Mol Biol. 2012;46:677–86.
30. Blanchard C, Mingler MK, McBride M, Putnam PE, Collins MH, Chang G, et al. Periostin facilitates eosinophil tissue infiltration in allergic lung and esophageal responses. Mucosal Immunol. 2008;1:289–96.
31. Noguchi T, Nakagome K, Kobayashi T, Uchida Y, Soma T, Nakamoto H, et al. Periostin upregulates the effector functions of eosinophils. J Allergy Clin Immunol. 2016;138:1449–52.
32. Wenzel SE. Asthma phenotypes: the evolution from clinical to molecular approaches. Nat Med. 2012;18:716–25.
33. Woodruff PG, Modrek B, Choy DF, Jia G, Abbas AR, Ellwanger A, et al. T-helper type 2-driven inflammation defines major subphenotypes of asthma. Am J Respir Crit Care Med. 2009;180:388–95.
34. Jia G, Erickson RW, Choy DF, Mosesova S, Wu LC, Solberg OD, et al. Periostin is a systemic biomarker of eosinophilic airway inflammation in asthmatic patients. J Allergy Clin Immunol. 2012;130:647–54.
35. Matsusaka M, Fukunaga K, Kabata H, Izuhara K, Asano K, Betsuyaku T. Subphenotypes of type 2 severe asthma in adults. J Allergy Clin Immunol Pract. 2018;6:274–6.
36. James A, Janson C, Malinovschi A, Holweg C, Alving K, Ono J, et al. Serum periostin relates to type-2 inflammation and lung function in asthma: data from the large population-based cohort Swedish GA(2)LEN. Allergy. 2017;72:1753–60.
37. Hinks TS, Brown T, Lau LC, Rupani H, Barber C, Elliott S, et al. Multidimensional endotyping in patients with severe asthma reveals inflammatory heterogeneity in matrix metalloproteinases and chitinase 3-like protein 1. J Allergy Clin Immunol. 2016;138:61–75.
38. Nagasaki T, Matsumoto H, Kanemitsu Y, Izuhara K, Tohda Y, Horiguchi T, et al. Using exhaled nitric oxide and serum periostin as a composite marker to identify severe/steroid-insensitive asthma. Am J Respir Crit Care Med. 2014;190:1449–52.
39. Nagasaki T, Matsumoto H, Kanemitsu Y, Izuhara K, Tohda Y, Kita H, et al. Integrating longitudinal information on pulmonary function and inflammation using asthma phenotypes. J Allergy Clin Immunol. 2014;133:1474–7.
40. Kato G, Takahashi K, Izuhara K, Komiya K, Kimura S, Hayashi S. Markers that can reflect asthmatic activity before and after reduction of inhaled corticosteroids: a pilot study. Biomark Insights. 2013;8:97–105.
41. Matsumoto H. Serum periostin: a novel biomarker for asthma management. Allergol Int. 2014;63:153–60.
42. Izuhara K, Matsumoto H, Ohta S, Ono J, Arima K, Ogawa M. Recent developments regarding periostin in bronchial asthma. Allergol Int. 2015;64(Suppl):S3–S10.
43. Corren J, Lemanske RF, Hanania NA, Korenblat PE, Parsey MV, Arron JR, et al. Lebrikizumab treatment in adults with asthma. N Engl J Med. 2011;365:1088–98.
44. Hanania NA, Korenblat P, Chapman KR, Bateman ED, Kopecky P, Paggiaro P, et al. Efficacy and safety of lebrikizumab in patients with uncontrolled asthma (LAVOLTA I and LAVOLTA II): replicate, phase 3, randomised, double-blind, placebo-controlled trials. Lancet Respir Med. 2016;4:781–96.

45. Brightling CE, Chanez P, Leigh R, O'Byrne PM, Korn S, She D, et al. Efficacy and safety of tralokinumab in patients with severe uncontrolled asthma: a randomised, double-blind, placebo-controlled, phase 2b trial. Lancet Respir Med. 2015;3:692–701.
46. Simpson EL, Bieber T, Guttman-Yassky E, Beck LA, Blauvelt A, Cork MJ, et al. Two phase 3 trials of dupilumab versus placebo in atopic dermatitis. N Engl J Med. 2016;376:1090–1.
47. Wenzel S, Castro M, Corren J, Maspero J, Wang L, Zhang B, et al. Dupilumab efficacy and safety in adults with uncontrolled persistent asthma despite use of medium-to-high-dose inhaled corticosteroids plus a long-acting β2 agonist: a randomised double-blind placebo-controlled pivotal phase 2b dose-ranging trial. Lancet. 2016;388:31–44.
48. Hanania NA, Wenzel S, Rosen K, Hsieh HJ, Mosesova S, Choy DF, et al. Exploring the effects of omalizumab in allergic asthma: an analysis of biomarkers in the EXTRA study. Am J Respir Crit Care Med. 2013;187:804–11.
49. Tajiri T, Matsumoto H, Gon Y, Ito R, Hashimoto S, Izuhara K, et al. Utility of serum periostin and free IgE levels in evaluating responsiveness to omalizumab in patients with severe asthma. Allergy. 2016;71:1472–9.

Chapter 8
Clinical Application of the Forced Oscillation Technique (FOT)

Toshihiro Shirai

Abstract The forced oscillation technique (FOT) is a noninvasive method for measurement of respiratory system resistance (Rrs) and reactance (Xrs) during tidal breathing, which avoids the requirement for forced expiration (as in spirometry). Its clinical application has progressed worldwide with the spread of commercially available broadband frequency FOT devices, including MostGraph and impulse oscillometry (IOS). An increasing number of reports have demonstrated the usefulness of FOT in the management of asthma and COPD. Rrs, especially Rrs at 5 Hz (R5), is a marker of airway caliber, i.e., airway narrowing. Since the changes in FOT parameters are generally greater than the changes in spirometry, the FOT may be useful in airway reversibility testing to diagnose asthma. By using both Rrs and Xrs, it is possible to differentiate asthma from COPD, particularly when combined with the characteristic colored 3D images produced by MostGraph. The FOT is not a surrogate test for spirometry but should be used complementarily. Furthermore, there is a need to establish reference values and provide interpretations of measured data.

Keywords Forced oscillation technique · Respiratory reactance · Respiratory resistance

8.1 Introduction

The forced oscillation technique (FOT) is a noninvasive method for measurement of lung mechanics [1, 2]. Forced oscillations are applied to the airway opening from the mouth to derive respiratory system impedance (Zrs), the spectral relationship between the resultant pressure and airflow. The real aspect of impedance is the

---

T. Shirai (✉)
Department of Respiratory Medicine, Shizuoka General Hospital, Shizuoka, Japan
e-mail: toshihiro-shirai@i.shizuoka-pho.jp

A. Yokoyama (ed.), *Advances in Asthma*, Respiratory Disease Series: Diagnostic Tools and Disease Managements, https://doi.org/10.1007/978-981-13-2790-2_8

respiratory system resistance (Rrs), whereas the imaginary aspect is the respiratory system reactance (Xrs), which is considered to reflect the elastic and inertial properties of the lung. Recently, clinical application of the broadband frequency FOT for measurement of lung function has progressed with the spread of commercially available FOT devices, including MostGraph (Chest M.I. Co. Ltd., Tokyo, Japan) and impulse oscillometry (IOS) (MasterScreen IOS; Jaeger, Hoechberg, Germany). An increasing number of studies have examined the usefulness of the FOT in the evaluation or management of obstructive lung diseases, including asthma and COPD. Forced oscillations can be superimposed on tidal breathing, thereby avoiding the need for any special breathing maneuver or noticeable interference with respiration. The FOT provides more information regarding the lung than can be obtained by forced expiration (spirometry). If reference values and proper interpretation of the measured data can be established, then this technique will be useful in older patients who experience difficulty in performing spirometry, as well as in young children who cannot cooperate with the maneuver. In this chapter, the author describes the role of the FOT in the diagnosis of asthma, according to the key features of the Japanese guidelines for adult asthma 2017 [3].

8.2 Measurements and Interpretation of the FOT

As the standard recommendations for measurements of the FOT are described elsewhere [1, 2], a few important points are shown here (Table 8.1).

Zrs is defined as the complex ratio of pressure to flow at the mouth and consists of Rrs and Xrs with the following relationship: $(Zrs)^2 = (Rrs)^2 + (Xrs)^2$.

Rrs indicates the total resistance of the respiratory system, including airway resistance (Raw), respiratory tissue resistance (Rti), and chest wall resistance (Rcw). Raw is a major portion of the Rrs; thus, Rrs, especially at 5 Hz (R5), is frequently interpreted as an index of airway caliber. Although both R5 and forced expiratory volume in 1 second (FEV1) are indices of airway obstruction, Rrs and FEV1 are not necessarily identical; however, they are closely related. Rrs at 20 Hz (R20) also correlates with FEV1 in asthma but more weakly than R5 [4, 5]. The difference between R5 and R20 (R5-R20) has been frequently used as a representative marker for the frequency dependence in FOT. In a previous study, R5-R20, particularly in the inspiratory phase, correlated with both %FEV1 and the N_2 phase III slope of single-breath N_2 washout (delta N_2), suggesting that R5-R20 exhibited a specific relationship with airway obstruction and ventilation inhomogeneity [5]. Some researchers have interpreted R5-R20 as peripheral airway resistance because they consider R5 and R20 to reflect the total and central airway resistances, respectively [6, 7]. However, those hypotheses of R5-R20 as peripheral resistance do not arise from any physiological basis, and there is no statement in any official guidelines that supports this interpretation. In addition, high R5-R20 values are physiologically detected in children mainly because of upper airway mechanics [8].

Table 8.1 Summary of the measurements and interpretation of forced oscillation technique (FOT)

Measurements
• Cheek support by an operator, not by the subject himself/herself, results in lower Rrs and smaller Xrs values for the patients
• Slow breathing (0.7-fold respiratory rate) causes higher Rrs values, whereas greater tidal breathing (1.5-fold tidal volume) causes higher Rrs and greater (more negative) Xrs values
Interpretation of the measured data
• Careful attention is required for both Rrs and Xrs values
• Data should be compared among whole-breath, inspiratory, and expiratory phases and the differences compared between inspiratory and expiratory phases
• Rrs, especially R5, reflects airway caliber
• R5-R20 is an indicator of the frequency dependence of Rrs, which is presumed to reflect ventilation inhomogeneity
• Do not use R5-R20 as a sole measurement approach
• X5, Fres, and ALX reflect abnormalities in the lung parenchyma or airways
• Compare R5 and Xrs with FEV1
• ΔX5 reflects the expiratory flow limitation, a major determinant of dynamic hyperinflation and exercise limitation
• The FOT may be useful during the bronchial reversibility test
• There is no relationship with fractional exhaled nitric oxide
• The FOT parameters may improve despite a lack of changes in spirometry
• Minimal clinically important differences have not yet been established
• The FOT is not a surrogate test for spirometry but should be used complementarily

ALX low-frequency reactance area, *Δ* difference between the inspiratory and expiratory phases, *FEV1* forced expiratory volume in 1 s, *FOT* forced oscillation technique, *Fres* resonant frequency, *Rrs* respiratory system resistance, *R5 and R20* Rrs at 5 Hz and 20 Hz, respectively, *R5-R20* the difference between R5 and R20, *X5* Xrs at 5 Hz, *Xrs* respiratory system reactance

Xrs is presumed to reflect the summation of elastic and inertial properties. It is negative at a low frequency and positive at a high frequency. The point at which Xrs = 0 is referred to as a resonant frequency (Fres), where elasticity and inertia balance each other. Generally, more elastic properties are associated with more negative Xrs values, whereas more inertial properties are associated with more positive Xrs values. Fres and Xrs at 5 Hz (X5) are frequently used as representative markers for Xrs. The low-frequency reactance area (ALX), which is the integral of X5 to the Fres, is also used. In patients with asthma, these three parameters were shown to significantly correlate with FEV1 and delta N_2, suggesting that may serve as other markers of airway obstruction and ventilator inhomogeneity [5, 9]. Although there are some differences in the details, the strongest correlation is generally found between Fres and FEV1 in both asthma and COPD [4, 5].

Oscillatory indices are expressed as the mean values of the whole data (whole-breath) and of each phase as inspiration or expiration. The difference between the inspiratory and expiratory phases (Δ) is also frequently used. Those basic indices can be easily obtained using either IOS or MostGraph. In addition, the latter software visualizes the time course as well as the absolute values in colored 3D graphics; this approach is suitable for both medical staff members and patients to understand various respiratory conditions, such as bronchoconstriction in asthma or the effects of treatment [10].

A comparative study using phantom models found that the measured values were closely consistent with, but not identical to, more negative Xrs values in IOS, rather than those in MostGraph [11]. Reference values of MostGraph and IOS are available for Japanese adults [12, 13]. However, more extensive reference values are needed. A summary of the interpretation of the FOT is shown in Table 8.1.

8.3 Key Features of the Diagnosis of Adult Asthma and the Role of the FOT

The role of the FOT in the diagnosis of adult asthma is discussed according to the key features of the Japanese guidelines for adult asthma 2017 (Table 8.2) [3].

8.3.1 Recurrence of Paroxysmal Dyspnea, Wheezing, Chest Tightness, and Cough (Particularly at Night and in the Early Morning)

A study using an in-house FOT system found that dyspnea (Borg scale) during a methacholine challenge was related to the increase in inspiratory R5 during mild bronchoconstriction (FEV1 decrease: <15%) [14]. Concerning the quality of life in asthmatic patients, a study using IOS found that R20, X5, and dose of inhaled

Table 8.2 Key features of the diagnosis of adult asthma [3]

1. Recurrence of paroxysmal dyspnea, wheezing, chest tightness, and cough (particularly at night and in the early morning)
2. Reversible airflow limitation
3. Airway hyperresponsiveness
4. Atopy
5. Airway inflammation
6. Differential diagnosis
a. Upper respiratory tract diseases: laryngitis, epiglottitis, vocal cord dysfunction
b. Proximal respiratory tract diseases: endotracheal tumor, foreign body aspiration, tracheomalacia, endobronchial tuberculosis
c. Diseases of the bronchus and alveolar regions: chronic obstructive pulmonary disease
d. Cardiovascular diseases: congestive heart failure, pulmonary thromboembolism
e. Cough induced by medicines, such as angiotensin-converting enzyme inhibitors
f. Other causes: spontaneous pneumothorax, hyperventilation syndrome, and psychogenic cough

Items 1, 2, 3, and 6 are important for diagnosis
Items 4 and 5, in combination with symptoms, support the diagnosis of asthma
Item 5 is typically indicative of eosinophilia

corticosteroid (ICS), but not FEV1, were significantly associated with scores on the Asthma Quality of Life Questionnaire in multiple regression analyses [15]. In patients with cough-variant asthma, cough, R5, and Xrs significantly improved, but not FEV1, following treatment with an ICS/long-acting β_2-agonist (LABA) combination, suggesting that R5 and Xrs may reflect mild bronchoconstriction in cough-variant asthma [16]. Home monitoring of inspiratory R5, using a monofrequency FOT device, was useful to diagnose asthma and predict acute deterioration of airway function, demonstrating the ability of the FOT to detect variable airway narrowing [17].

8.3.2 Reversible Airflow Limitation

The FOT is often used together with spirometry in airway reversibility tests. Overall, Rrs decreases after bronchodilation, especially at low frequencies [1]. Figure 8.1 shows a representative case of asthma who fulfilled the American Thoracic Society

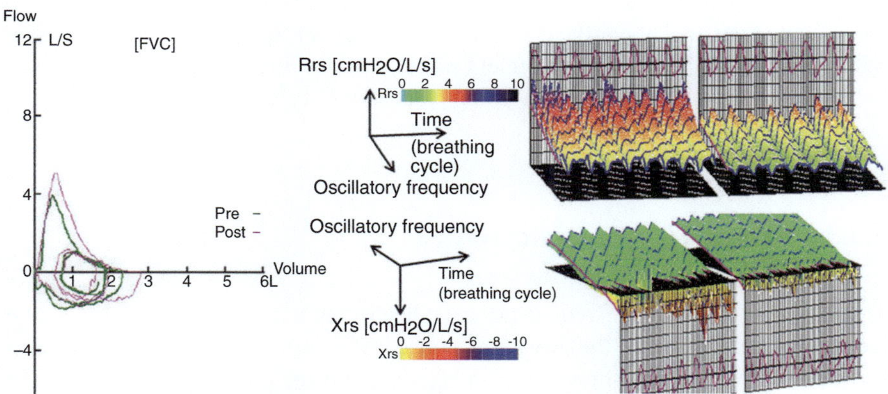

	Pre	Post	% Change
FVC [L]	2.49	2.95	+18.5 (460 mL)
FEV1 [L]	1.59	1.84	+15.7 (250 mL)
R5 [cmH20/L/s]	4.78	3.13	+34.5
R20 [cmH20/L/s]	3.50	2.50	+28.6
R5-R20 [cmH20/L/s]	1.28	0.63	+50.8
X5 [cmH20/L/s]	−1.43	−0.59	+58.7
Fres [Hz]	13.96	8.67	+37.9
ALX [cmH20/L/s * Hz]	7.92	2.12	+73.2

Fig. 8.1 Changes in pre- and post-bronchodilator spirometric and forced oscillatory parameters in a patient with asthma in airway reversibility testing. Oscillatory parameters of MostGraph are expressed as whole-breath values. *ALX* low-frequency reactance area, *FEV₁* forced expiratory volume in 1 s, *Fres* resonant frequency, *FVC* forced vital capacity, *Rrs* respiratory system resistance, *R5 and R20* Rrs at 5 Hz and 20 Hz, respectively, *R5-R20* the difference between R5 and R20, *Xrs* respiratory system reactance, *X5* Xrs at 5 Hz

criteria, which suggest a significant post-bronchodilator FEV1 and/or forced vital capacity response of ≥200 mL and 12% improvement from baseline [18]. Since the changes in FOT parameters are generally greater than changes observed in spirometry, an approximate 30% change in R5, for example, together with the change in color 3D images demonstrated by MostGraph, suggests the presence of airway reversibility and a diagnosis of asthma. Although the range of the Rrs response to bronchodilators in children is reported to be 20–40% [19], those values in adults have not been established. An occasional lack of correlation between spirometric and forced oscillatory parameter changes makes it difficult to establish such values. In addition, of course, airway reversibility is sometimes present in patients with COPD. The difference in R5 and X5 between pre- and post-bronchodilator inhalation using MostGraph was significantly greater in asthmatic than in nonasthmatic children [8]. The receiver operator characteristic (ROC) curve analyses revealed that the difference in X5 (cutoff value: 0.46 $cmH_2O/L/s$) was the best predictor for FEV1 reversibility.

The ability of FOT parameters to predict an improvement in FEV1 after ICS/LABA combination treatment was investigated in 31 untreated patients with asthma [20]. In multivariate logistic regression analyses, >10% change in FEV1 was independently predicted by R5 (adjusted odds ratio 15.9). The ROC curve analyses also revealed that the area under the curve (AUC) was higher for R5 (0.731) than for any other parameters. To detect a treatment effect or daily fluctuations, minimal clinically important differences in FOT parameters should be established.

8.3.3 Airway Hyperresponsiveness

The values of Rrs at lower frequencies have been shown to be reliable and sensitive indices for assessment of the airway response during clinical airway hyperresponsiveness testing [1]. In a study using an apparatus for the continuous methacholine inhalation method, with simultaneous measurement of Rrs at 3 Hz (Astograph; Chest M.I. Co. Ltd., Tokyo, Japan), FEV1 was also measured at baseline and immediately after a twofold increase of Rrs [21]. In that study, the mean change in FEV1 was −19.3%, suggesting a parallel change between FEV1 and Rrs. A study evaluated the complementary roles of fractional exhaled nitric oxide (FeNO) and FOT (MostGraph) to predict airway hyperresponsiveness in adult stable asthmatic patients who were taking ICS [22]; the results showed that a combined R5 >3.30 $cmH_2O/L/s$ and FeNO >37.8 ppb could predict 65.7% positivity in the airway hyperresponsiveness test (Japanese Society of Allergology standard method). Another unpublished study investigated whether FOT (MostGraph) could predict airway hyperresponsiveness measured by using Astograph [23]. The ROC analysis revealed that the AUC of a combination inspiratory R5 and body mass index was 0.821, suggesting that FOT may be useful to predict airway hyperresponsiveness. An adult study using IOS also revealed that asthmatic patients showed higher

R5-R20 and more negative X5, compared with subjects with asymptomatic bronchial hyperresponsiveness, as well as healthy controls [24].

8.3.4 *Atopy*

There is no relationship between atopy and the FOT.

8.3.5 *Airway Inflammation*

As stated in Chap. 9 of this book, IL-13- or IL-4-related eosinophilic airway inflammation can be detected via FeNO measurements. There is no correlation between FeNO and Rrs or Xrs [5, 25]. However, weak correlations were found between alveolar nitric oxide concentration (CANO), a marker that reflects peripheral airway or alveolar inflammation, and whole-breath R5-R20, X5, and ALX, using IOS [25, 26]. In contrast, another study using MostGraph found significant correlations between CANO and ΔX5, ΔFres, and ΔALX [5]. Since ΔXrs, especially ΔX5, is considered to reflect expiratory flow limitation, these findings may suggest a relationship between peripheral airway obstruction and reduced CANO. In addition, the discrepancy may be explained by the difference in the devices used and the two-sidedness of FeNO and CANO, i.e., asthma exacerbation causes higher values, whereas bronchoconstriction sometimes causes lower values. Further studies are needed to establish those findings.

8.3.6 *Differential Diagnosis*

8.3.6.1 Vocal Cord Dysfunction

A case of vocal cord dysfunction, which was identified by laryngoscopy, was reported [27]. By using an in-house monofrequency FOT, the paradoxical adduction of the vocal cords was revealed by breathing-related changes in the Rrs, which showed prominent increase during inspiration and a large positive difference between inspiration and expiration.

8.3.6.2 Relapsing Polychondritis

Patients with relapsing polychondritis and airway stenosis have difficulty in performing conventional spirometry that requires maximum forced expiration. A case was reported in which a combination of three-dimensional computed tomography and FOT (MostGraph) was useful for assessing airway stenosis while reducing the burden of repeated spirometry. The Rrs exhibited high values at the time of diagnosis, resembling features of COPD [28].

8.3.6.3 COPD

As stated earlier, the colored 3D graphic images produced by MostGraph exhibit an advantage in that they visualize both frequency and respiratory cycle dependence. The images can generally be classified into three types (Fig. 8.2) [4, 10]. The Rrs of the first pattern demonstrates high values during the expiratory phases (blue or black at the top, i.e., ≥6 $cmH_2O/L/s$) and low values during the inspiratory phases (green or yellow at the bottom, i.e., approximately 2 $cmH_2O/L/s$) with a marked frequency dependence (increasing at lower frequencies) and respiratory cycle dependence (greater differences between the expiratory and inspiratory phases). Xrs shows greater (more negative) values (occasionally blue at the bottom, i.e., <−6 $cmH_2O/L/s$). This pattern is typically found in patients with COPD but can be found in those with severe or uncontrolled asthma (Fig. 8.2, left panel). The Rrs of the second pattern exhibits moderately high Rrs throughout the entire frequency and respiratory cycle (yellow, orange, or red, i.e., approximately 4 $cmH_2O/L/s$) with slight frequency and respiratory cycle dependence and Xrs changes (yellow); this pattern is typically found in patients with asthma but can be found in those with COPD and in healthy controls (Fig. 8.2, middle panel). The Rrs of the third pattern shows low Rrs (green, i.e., <2 $cmH_2O/L/s$) and Xrs (yellow) values with few within-breath changes; this pattern is usually found in healthy controls but can be found in patients with mild or controlled asthma and sometimes in those with COPD (Fig. 8.2, right panel). Roughly speaking, in clinical practice, it is possible to differentiate asthma from COPD based on these characteristic 3D images. A previous study using MostGraph revealed that ΔX5 contributed significantly to the

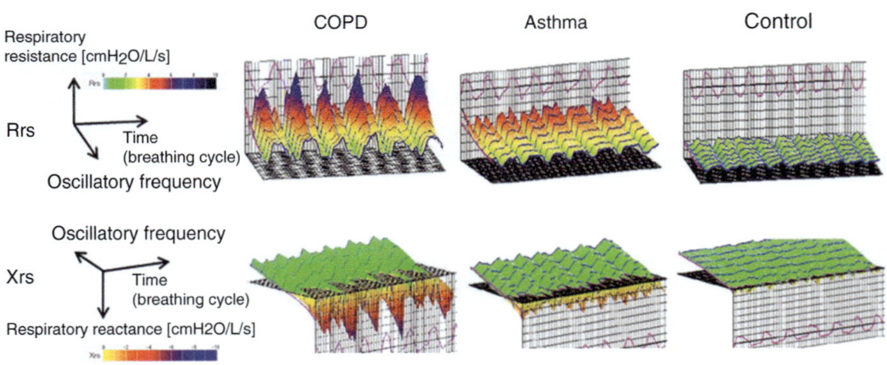

Fig. 8.2 Colored three-dimensional images of respiratory system resistance (Rrs) and reactance (Xrs) in each representative subject. *Exp* expiratory, *insp* inspiratory

differentiation between asthma and COPD, independent of age, gender, body weight, and spirometry [4].

8.4 Conclusion

The FOT is a lung function test to detect airway narrowing that does not require forced expiration, as in spirometry. Since the changes in FOT parameters are generally greater than those observed in spirometry, the FOT may be useful in airway reversibility testing. By using both resistance and reactance, it is possible to differentiate asthma from COPD. Thus, the FOT is not a surrogate test for spirometry but should be used complementarily.

References

1. Oostveen E, Macleod D, Lorino H, Farré R, Hantos Z, Desager K, et al. The forced oscillation technique in clinical practice: methodology, recommendations and future developments. Eur Respir J. 2003;22:1026–41.
2. Shirai T, Kurosawa H. Clinical application of the forced oscillation technique. Intern Med. 2016;55(6):559–66. https://doi.org/10.2169/internalmedicine.55.5876.
3. Ichinose M, Sugiura H, Nagase H, Yamaguchi M, Inoue H, Sagara H, Tamaoki J, Tohda Y, Munakata M, Yamauchi K, Ohta K, Japanese Society of Allergology. Japanese guidelines for adult asthma 2017. Allergol Int. 2017;66:163–89. https://doi.org/10.1016/j.alit.2016.12.005.
4. Mori K, Shirai T, Mikamo M, Shishido Y, Akita T, Morita S, et al. Colored 3-dimensional analyses of respiratory resistance and reactance in COPD and asthma. COPD. 2011;8:456–63. https://doi.org/10.3109/15412555.2011.626818.
5. Shirai T, Mori K, Mikamo M, Shishido Y, Akita T, Morita S, et al. Respiratory mechanics and peripheral airway inflammation and dysfunction in asthma. Clin Exp Allergy. 2013;43:521–6. https://doi.org/10.1016/j.anai.2012.02.007.
6. Shi Y, Aledia AS, Galant SP, George SC. Peripheral airway impairment measured by oscillometry predicts loss of asthma control in children. J Allergy Clin Immunol. 2013;131:718–23. https://doi.org/10.1016/j.jaci.2012.09.022.
7. Bickel S, Popler J, Lesnick B, Eid N. Impulse oscillometry. Interpretation and practical applications. Chest. 2014;146:841–7. https://doi.org/10.1378/chest.13-1875.
8. Murakami K, Habukawa C, Kurosawa H, Takemura T. Evaluation of airway responsiveness using colored three-dimensional analyses of a new forced oscillation technique in controlled asthmatic and nonasthmatic children. Respir Investig. 2014;52:57–64. https://doi.org/10.1016/j.resinv.2013.07.003.
9. Shirai T, Mori K, Tsuchiya T, Suda T. Resonant frequency as a predictor of phase 3 slope of nitrogen single-breath washout in asthma. Ann Allergy Asthma Immunol. 2015;115:73–4. https://doi.org/10.1016/j.anai.2015.05.003.
10. Shirai T, Mori K, Mikamo M, Shishido Y, Akita T, Morita S, et al. Usefulness of colored 3D imaging of respiratory impedance in asthma. Allergy, Asthma Immunol Res. 2013;5:322–8. https://doi.org/10.4168/aair.2013.5.5.322.
11. Tanimura K, Hirai T, Sato S, Hasegawa K, Muro S, Kurosawa H, et al. Comparison of two devices for respiratory impedance measurement using a forced oscillation technique: basic study using phantom models. J Physiol Sci. 2014;64:377–82. https://doi.org/10.1007/s12576-014-0329-4.

12. Abe Y, Shibata Y, Igarashi A, Inoue S, Sato K, Sato M, et al. Reference values of MostGraph measures for middle-aged and elderly Japanese individuals who participated in annual health checkups. Respir Investig. 2016;54:148–55. https://doi.org/10.1016/j.resinv.2015.12.004.
13. Shiota S, Katoh M, Fujii M, Aoki S, Matsuoka R, Fukuchi Y. Predictive equations and the reliability of the impulse oscillatory system in Japanese adult subjects. Respirology. 2005;10:310–5.
14. Antonelli A, Crimi E, Gobbi A, Torchio R, Gulotta C, Dellaca R, et al. Mechanical correlates of dyspnea in bronchial asthma. Physiol Rep. 2013;1:e00166. https://doi.org/10.1002/phy2.166.
15. Takeda T, Oga T, Niimi A, Matsumoto H, Ito I, Yamaguchi M, et al. Relationship between small airway function and health status, dyspnea and disease control in asthma. Respiration. 2010;80:120–6. https://doi.org/10.1159/000242113.
16. Watanabe H, Tanaka Y, Endo Y, Suzuki T, Noguchi R, Saigusa M, et al. Usefulness of the forced oscillation technique in the management of cough variant asthma. The 66th Annual Meeting of Japanese Society of Allergology. 2017, Tokyo.
17. Gulotta C, Suki B, Brusasco V, Pellegrino R, Gobbi A, Pedotti A, et al. Monitoring the temporal changes of respiratory resistance: a novel test for the management of asthma. Am J Respir Crit Care Med. 2012;185:1330–1.
18. American Thoracic Society. Standardization of spirometry, 1994 update. Am J Respir Crit Care Med. 1995;152:1107–36.
19. Beydon N, Davis SD, Lombardi E, Allen JL, Arets HG, Aurora P, et al. An official American Thoracic Society/European Respiratory Society statement: pulmonary function testing in preschool children. Am J Respir Crit Care Med. 2007;175:1304–45.
20. Akamatsu T, Shirai T, Shimoda Y, Suzuki T, Hayashi I, Noguchi R, et al. Forced oscillation technique as a predictor of FEV1 improvement in asthma. Respir Physiol Neurobiol. 2017;236:78–83. https://doi.org/10.1016/j.resp.2016.11.013.
21. Niimi A, Matsumoto H, Takemura M, Ueda T, Chin K, Mishima M. Relationship of airway wall thickness to airway sensitivity and airway reactivity in asthma. Am J Respir Crit Care Med. 2003;168:983–8.
22. Fukuhara M, Tsuburai T, Nakamura Y, Tomita Y, Hamada Y, Watai K, et al. The fraction of exhaled nitric oxide (FeNO) and forced oscillation technique (FOT) can predict bronchial hyperresponsiveness against acetylcholine in treated asthmatics. Arerugi. 2017;66:42–9. https://doi.org/10.15036/arerugi.66.42.
23. Akamatsu T, Tanaka Y, Watanabe H, Endo Y, Shimoda Y, Suzuki T, et al. Forced oscillation technique as a predictor of airway hyperresponsiveness in asthma. The Congress of European Respiratory Society. 2016, London.
24. Boudewijin IM, Telenga ED, van der Wiel E, van der Molen T, Schiphof L, Ten Hacken NH, et al. Less small airway dysfunction in asymptomatic bronchial hyperresponsiveness than in asthma. Allergy. 2013;68:1419–26. https://doi.org/10.1111/all.12242.
25. Matsumoto H, Niimi A, Jinnai M, Nakaji H, Takeda T, Oguma T, et al. Association of alveolar nitric oxide levels with pulmonary function and its reversibility in stable asthma. Respiration. 2011;81:311–7. https://doi.org/10.1159/000319566.
26. Williamson PA, Clearie K, Menzies D, Vaidyanathan S, Lipworth BJ. Assessment of small-airways disease using alveolar nitric oxide and impulse oscillometry in asthma and COPD. Lung. 2011;189:121–9. https://doi.org/10.1007/s00408-010-9275-y.
27. Ioan I, Marchal F, Coffinet L, Coutier L, Bonabel C, Demoulin B, et al. Breathing-related changes of respiratory resistance in vocal cord dysfunction. Respirology. 2016;21:1134–6. https://doi.org/10.1111/resp.12735.
28. Shimizu Y, Kamiyoshihara M, Okajo J, Ishii Y, Takise A. Tracheobronchial stenosis evaluated by inspiratory and expiratory three-dimensional computed tomography and impulse oscillation with three-dimensional color imaging in a patient with relapsing polychondritis. J Biol Regul Homeost Agents. 2014;28:325–31.

Chapter 9
Diagnostic Value of Fractional Exhaled Nitric Oxide (FeNO)

Kazuto Matsunaga

Abstract Asthma is a heterogeneous disease, usually characterized by chronic inflammation of the airways. Fractional nitric oxide (NO) concentration in exhaled air (FeNO) is recognized as a noninvasive biomarker of eosinophilic inflammation in the lower respiratory tract. Presence of airway inflammation in addition to respiratory symptoms that are suggestive of asthma supports a diagnosis of asthma. This chapter provides recent topics pertaining to asthma including the mechanism of production of NO in the airway, methods of and interpretations in measuring FeNO, and the role of exhaled NO measurement in making diagnosis of asthma and differentiating asthma from chronic obstructive pulmonary disease (COPD).

Keywords Asthma · Airway inflammation · COPD · Exhaled nitric oxide · Type 2

Abbreviations

ACO	Asthma-COPD overlap
COPD	Chronic obstructive pulmonary disease
eNOS	Endothelial nitric oxide synthase
FeNO	Fractional nitric oxide concentration in exhaled air
FEV1	Forced expiratory volume in one second
FVC	Forced vital capacity
iNOS	Inducible nitric oxide synthase
NO	Nitric oxide
nNOS	Neuronal nitric oxide synthase
ROS	Reactive oxygen species

K. Matsunaga (✉)
Department of Respiratory Medicine and Infectious Disease, Graduate School of Medicine, Yamaguchi University, Ube, Japan
e-mail: kazmatsu@yamaguchi-u.ac.jp

A. Yokoyama (ed.), *Advances in Asthma*, Respiratory Disease Series: Diagnostic Tools and Disease Managements, https://doi.org/10.1007/978-981-13-2790-2_9

9.1 Introduction

Although asthma is a disease showing various symptoms and pathologies, chronic airway inflammation is a consistent feature of the disease and the primary target of its treatment. Airway inflammation has traditionally been assessed using sputum and/or biopsy tissue samples, but such assessments are disadvantageous due to patient invasiveness and poor rapidity of test results. Exhaled nitric oxide (NO) that allows noninvasive and real-time measurement reflects eosinophilic inflammation in the lower respiratory tract and therefore, useful for making a diagnosis of asthma and predicting steroid responsiveness [1–3]. Moreover, since changes in FeNO levels during anti-inflammatory treatment correlate with improvement in symptoms, airflow limitation, and airway hyperresponsiveness [4–6], exhaled NO is expected to play an important role in monitoring of asthma and guide for its treatment. FeNO measurement as a biomarker to assess the airway inflammation has been covered by health insurance in Japan since 2013.

9.2 Measurement of Exhaled Nitric Oxide: Basic Aspects

In the human body, NO is produced by NO synthase (NOS) when L-arginine is converted to L-citrulline (Fig. 9.1). Three isoforms of NO have been identified to date, and their activation mechanism, expression patterns, and intracellular localization have been

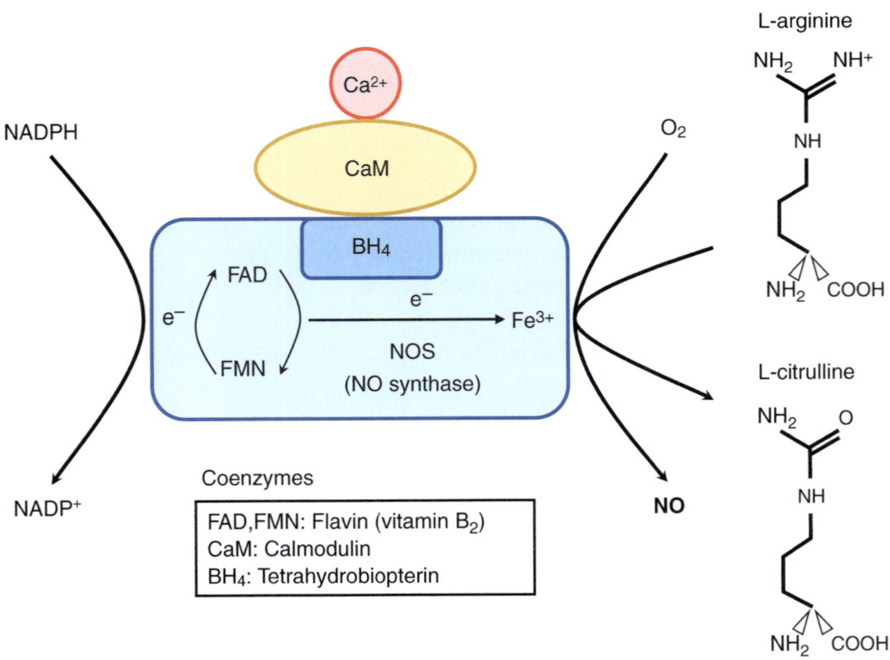

Fig. 9.1 Molecular mechanism of nitric oxide synthesis

Table 9.1 Isoforms of nitric oxide synthase and localization site in the airways

Isoform	Type 1 (nNOS)	Type 2 (iNOS)	Type 3 (eNOS)
Chromosome position	12q4.2	17q11.2-q12	7q35-q36
Molecular weight	160 kDa	130 kDa	133 kDa
Dependence of calmodulin	+	+	+
Dependence of calcium	+	–	+
Major expression site	Neuron	Macrophage	Endothelium
Localization site in the airways	Nerve fiber Airway epithelium Neutrophil	Macrophage Airway epithelium Fibroblast Vascular smooth muscle Vascular endothelium Neutrophil Mast cell Eosinophil	Vascular endothelium Airway epithelium Platelet

nNOS neuronal nitric oxide synthase, *iNOS* inducible nitric oxide synthase, *eNOS* endothelial nitric oxide synthase

characterized (Table 9.1). Neuronal NOS (nNOS) expressed in neurons and skeletal muscle cells as well as endothelial NOS (eNOS) expressed in vascular endothelial cells are constitutively expressed enzymes, which require increased Ca^{2+} level in the cytoplasm induced by stimulation with agonists (e.g., acetylcholine) for activation and are characterized by Ca^{2+}-dependent action for a short time. On the other hand, inducible NOS (iNOS) whose mRNA is synthesized by stimulation with inflammatory cytokines and endotoxins does not depend on Ca^{2+} levels after its production and produces larger quantities of NO for longer time than constitutively expressed NOS [1, 2].

Th2 cells, ILC2 cells, and mast cells that produce inflammatory type 2 cytokines such as interleukin (IL)-4, IL-5, and IL-13 are activated in patients with asthma. IL-4 and IL-13 induce synthesis of iNOS in airway epithelial cells via transcription of STAT-6, resulting in production of a large quantities of NO [7]. Thus, higher level of NO is detected in the exhaled air from patients with asthma than that from healthy individuals [8]. In patients with asthma, FeNO correlates with the severity of eosinophilic airway inflammation determined using sputum or biopsy tissue samples. Therefore, exhaled NO measurement is regarded as "a noninvasive test to detect eosinophilic inflammation in the lower respiratory tract" [1–3]. Chronic obstructive pulmonary disease (COPD), an inflammatory airway disease like as asthma, however, is not associated with increased FeNO levels since NO is consumed by reactive oxygen species (ROS) locally in the airway of patients with COPD [8].

Measurement of exhaled NO requires standardization of measurement conditions since FeNO is affected by various factors including expiratory flow rate and mouth pressure. Recommendations for standardized procedures for measurement of exhaled NO were issued in 2005 by the American Thoracic Society (ATS) and European Respiratory Society (ERS) [1]. The main recommendations are as follows: (1) Since exhaled NO levels exhibit a significant dependence on expiratory flow rate, a constant expiratory flow rate of 50 mL/s should be achieved and maintained during measurement. (2)

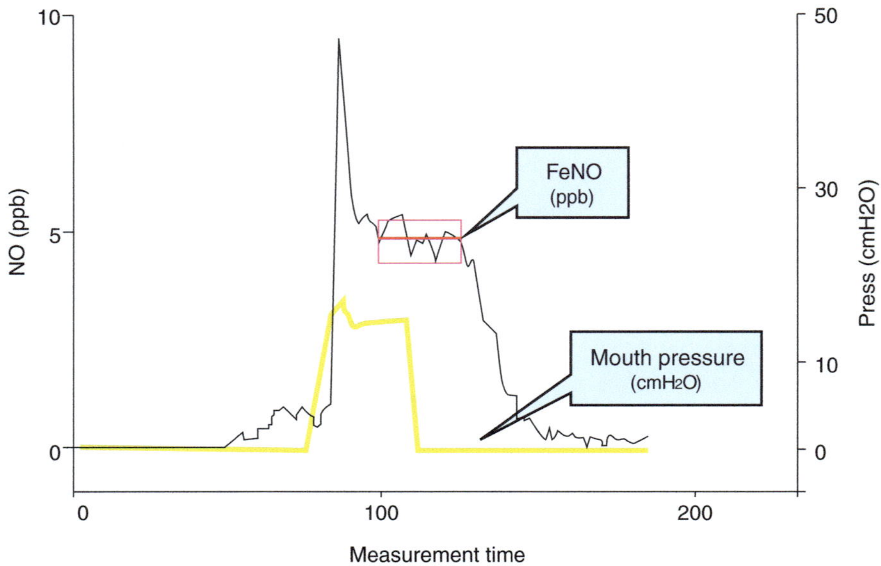

Fig. 9.2 Exhaled nitric oxide concentration and mouth pressure versus time for the single exhalation. This figure shows an early peak due to contamination with NO from the nasal cavity and dead space, followed by a certain NO plateau phase (red line). This plateau value should be regarded as an exhaled NO from the lower respiratory tract

Exhalation should be started at the point of total lung capacity. (3) The mouth pressure should be 5–15 cm H_2O to ensure closure of the velopharyngeal aperture and exclude contamination of the nasal NO (containing upper respiratory tract NO). (4) The exhaled NO profile versus time shows an early peak due to contamination with NO from the nasal cavity and dead space, followed by a certain NO plateau phase. This value is stable if an appropriate mouth pressure at expiration and a constant expiratory flow rate are ensured. This plateau value should be regarded as an exhaled NO from the lower respiratory tract (FeNO) (Fig. 9.2).

As of January 2018, three maintenance-free online devices for exhaled NO measurement have been approved for use under health insurance medical services in Japan: NIOX MINO® and NIOX VERO® from CHEST MI, Inc. and NObreath® from HARADA corporation.

9.3 Role of FeNO Measurement in the Diagnosis of Asthma

Diagnosis of asthma is based not only characteristic symptoms including paroxysmal wheezing that is likely to occur at night and in the early morning, dyspnea, and recurrent cough but also such physiological signs as reversible airflow limitation and increased airway hyperresponsiveness. An atopic predisposition and presence of airway inflammation (i.e., sputum eosinophilia and increased FeNO) usually support the diagnosis of asthma[3].

Clinical application of FeNO measurement requires establishment of specific normal ranges or cutoff values. A study to establish a normal range in Japanese revealed the mean FeNO level in healthy adults of 15 ppb and the statistically estimated upper limit of normal of 37 ppb [9]. In adults, such factors as gender, height, and body mass index (BMI) had no statistically significant effects on FeNO levels [9]. In another study, FeNO levels were compared between healthy adults with normal lung function and without respiratory symptoms and steroid-naive asthmatic patients with respiratory symptoms suggesting asthma who showed significant bronchodilator reversibility and/or increased airway hyperresponsiveness to determine a FeNO cutoff value for diagnosis of asthma [10]. FeNO levels were significantly higher in patients with asthma than in healthy volunteers, and a cutoff value to distinguish these two populations was calculated to be 22 ppb with a sensitivity of 91% and a specificity of 84% [10]. The area under the curve (AUC) from a receiver operating characteristic (ROC) analysis was 0.90, indicating that an FeNO level of ≥22 ppb in addition to presence of respiratory symptoms is associated with a high likelihood of asthma [10]. On the other hand, the sensitivity and specificity for diagnosis of asthma of a cutoff value of 37 ppb, the upper limit of normal [9], were 52% and 99%, respectively. Therefore, the use of this value should be associated with a low false-positive rate and is good for catching actual cases of asthma (high specificity). It should be noted, however, that the use of this cutoff value is associated with a high risk of missing cases of asthma (low sensitivity) (Fig. 9.3).

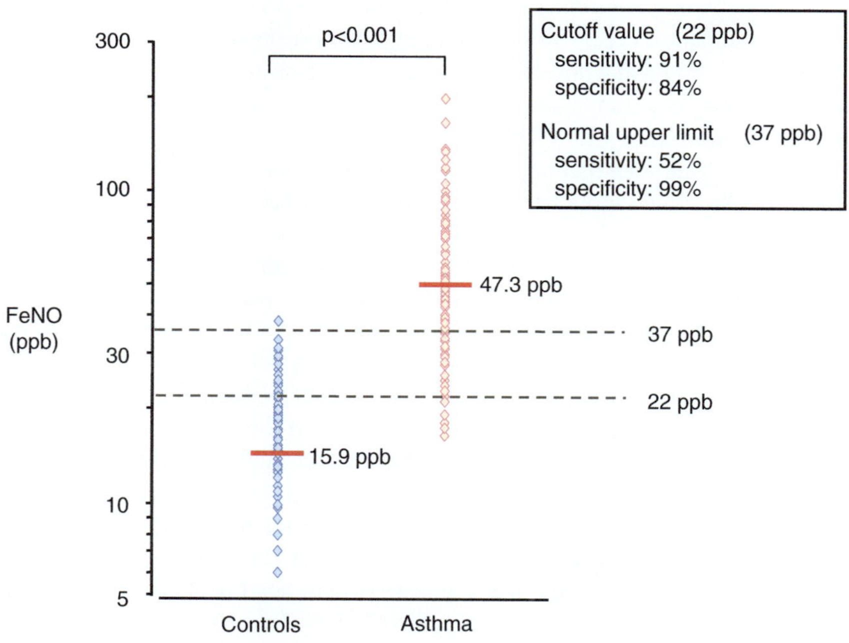

Fig. 9.3 Reference values of FeNO to support the diagnosis of asthma. Scatter plot of the FeNO levels in control subjects ($n = 224$) and asthmatic patients ($n = 142$). The horizontal red bars indicated the mean value for each group. The dotted lines indicated the cutoff value for asthma diagnosis (22 ppb) and the normal upper limit of Japanese healthy subjects (37 ppb), respectively

Additionally, multivariate analysis in the above two populations identified current smoking and allergic rhinitis as individual factors significantly affecting FeNO levels. Irrespective of asthma, individuals with rhinitis had significantly higher EeNO levels, and current smokers had significantly lower FeNO levels [10]. When the study subjects were divided into four subgroups according to current smoking status and concurrent rhinitis, subgroup analyses revealed cutoff values for diagnosis of asthma of 22 ppb in non-smokers without rhinitis, 28 ppb in non-smokers with rhinitis, 18 ppb in current smokers without rhinitis, and 22 ppb in current smokers with rhinitis. Although the cutoff value of FeNO varied depending on host factors, their sensitivity and specificity were high in all of the four subgroups, and the AUC was not lower than 0.85 in any subgroup, indicating that FeNO provides an adequately reliable complementary tool to support the diagnosis of asthma [10].

9.4 Exhaled NO Concentrations in Asthma and COPD

COPD, a disease characterized by persistent airflow limitation caused by pulmonary or respiratory tract injury mainly due to inhaled harmful particles such as tobacco, is of importance both in differentiation of asthma and as a complication of asthma [11]. Although both asthma and COPD are inflammatory airway disease, different types of inflammation are involved in them; asthma is characterized by eosinophilic and/or $CD4^+$ lymphocyte-mediated inflammation, while neutrophils and/or $CT8^+$ lymphocytes mainly contribute to inflammation in COPD [11, 12]. Assessment of airway inflammation is helpful for differentiation of asthma and COPD in patients for whom differential diagnosis is difficult only based on symptoms and physiological examination. In a study comparing age- and airflow limitation-matched patients with asthma and those with COPD, the FeNO level in patients with asthma was significantly higher than that in patients with COPD, and the sensitivity and specificity of the reported cutoff FeNO value for differential diagnosis (35 ppb) were 91% and 77%, respectively [12].

Some patients with asthma mainly complain of exertional dyspnea and show persistent airflow limitation that will not be normalized even after the inhalation of bronchodilator. On the other hand, some patients with COPD show bronchodilator reversibility even though their FEV_1 (forced expiratory volume in one second)/FVC (forced vital capacity) cannot be normalized with bronchodilators. Such patients that have both several features usually associated with asthma and several features usually associated with COPD and show persistent airflow limitation are currently called patients with asthma-COPD overlap (ACO) [11]. In Japanese guidelines [3], it is recommended that concurrent asthma should be considered and reflected in the treatment strategy for patients with COPD in whom at least one of the following is observed after excluding alternative diagnoses such as heart failure and lung cancer: paroxysmal dyspnea or wheezing, reversible airflow limitation, increased airway hyperresponsiveness, atopic predisposition, and any sign of airway inflammation such as sputum eosinophilia and increased FeNO level. Some patients with a clinical diagnosis of COPD show the type 2 molecular signatures (e.g., IL-4, IL-5, and IL-13) assessed by several biomarkers, such as immunoglobulin E, eosinophils in the blood or sputum, serum periostin, and FeNO [13–15]. Interestingly, presence of type 2 inflammation in COPD is strongly associated with responsiveness to steroid therapy [16, 17]. The mean FeNO level in patients with COPD was approximately 20 ppb, with a considerable highly variation [15]. It has been reported that approximately 16% of patients with COPD demonstrated high FeNO levels of at least 35 ppb which strongly suggested concurrent asthma from the viewpoint of inflammatory profile of the airway [15].

9.5 Conclusion

Measurement of exhaled NO may be affected not only by measurement conditions such as expiratory flow rate and mouth pressure but also by various host factors. Many recent studies, however, have shown that increased level of FeNO measured by standardized method is an important type 2 signature that supports the diagnosis of asthma. Assessment of airway inflammation using exhaled NO in addition to traditional assessments of symptoms and lung function is expected to allow further improvement of efficiency in management of chronic inflammatory airway diseases including asthma and COPD.

References

1. American Thoracic Society; European Respiratory Society. ATS/ERS recommendations for standardized procedures for the online and offline measurement of exhaled lower respiratory nitric oxide and nasal nitric oxide. Am J Respir Crit Care Med. 2005;171:912–30.
2. Dweik RA, Boggs PB, Erzurum SC, Irvin CG, Leigh MW, Lundberg JO, Olin AC, Plummer AL, Taylor DR, American Thoracic Society Committee on Interpretation of Exhaled Nitric Oxide Levels (FENO) for Clinical Applications. An official ATS clinical practice guideline: interpretation of exhaled nitric oxide levels (FeNO) for clinical applications. Am J Respir Crit Care Med. 2011;184:602–15.
3. Ichinose M, Sugiura H, Nagase H, Yamaguchi M, Inoue H, Sagara H, Tamaoki J, Tohda Y, Munakata M, Yamauchi K, Ohta K, Japanese Society of Allergy. Japanese guidelines for adult asthma. Allergol Int. 2017;66:163–89.
4. Ichinose M, Takahashi T, Sugiura H, Endoh N, Miura M, Mashito Y, Shirato K. Baseline airway hyperresponsiveness and its reversible component: role of airway inflammation and airway caliber. Eur Respir J. 2000;15:248–53.
5. Matsunaga K, Kawabata H, Hirano T, Sugiura H, Minakata Y, Ichnose M. Difference in time-course of improvement in asthma control measures between budesonide and budesonide/formoterol. Pulm Pharmacol Ther. 2013;26:189–94.
6. Matsunaga K, Hirano T, Akamatsu K, Minakata Y. Predictors for identifying the efficacy of systemic steroids on sustained exhaled nitric oxide elevation in severe asthma. Allergol Int. 2013;62:359–65.
7. Alving K, Malinovschi A. Basic aspects of exhaled nitric oxide. Eur Respir Mon. 2010;49:1–31.

8. Ichinose M, Sugiura H, Yamagata S, Koarai A, Shirato K. Increase in reactive nitrogen species production in chronic obstructive pulmonary disease airways. Am J Respir Crit Care Med. 2000;162:701–6.
9. Matsunaga K, Hirano T, Kawayama T, Tsuburai T, Nagase H, Aizawa H, Akiyama K, Ohta K, Ichinose M. Reference ranges for exhaled nitric oxide fraction in healthy Japanese adult population. Allergol Int. 2010;59:363–7.
10. Matsunaga K, Hirano T, Akamatsu K, Koarai A, Sugiura H, Minakata Y, Ichinose M. Exhaled nitric oxide cutoff values for asthma diagnosis according to rhinitis and smoking status in Japanese subjects. Allergol Int. 2011;60:331–7.
11. Global Initiative for Chronic Obstructive Lung Disease: Global strategy for the diagnosis, management, and prevention of chronic obstructive pulmonary disease, NHLBI/WHO workshop report 2017.
12. Fabbri LM, Romagnoli M, Corbetta L, Casoni G, Busljetic K, Turato G, Ligabue G, Ciaccia A, Saetta M, Papi A. Differences in airway inflammation in patients with fixed airflow obstruction due to asthma or chronic obstructive pulmonary disease. Am J Respir Crit Care Med. 2003;167:418–24.
13. McDonald VM, Higgins I, Wood LG, Gibson PG. Multidimensional assessment and tailored interventions for COPD: respiratory utopia or common sense? Thorax. 2013;68:691–4.
14. Konstantelou E, Papaioannou AI, Loukides S, Bartziokas K, Papaporfyriou A, Papatheodorou G, Bakakos P, Papiris S, Koulouris N, Kostikas K. Serum periostin in patients hospitalized for COPD exacerbations. Cytokine. 2017;93:51–6.
15. Tamada T, Sugiura H, Takahashi T, Matsunaga K, Kimura K, Katsumata U, Takekoshi D, Kikuchi T, Ohta K, Ichinose M. Biomarker-based detection of asthma-COPD overlap syndrome in COPD populations. Int J Chron Obstruct Pulmon Dis. 2015;10:2169–76.
16. Akamatsu K, Matsunaga K, Sugiura H, Koarai A, Hirano T, Minakata Y, Ichinose M. Improvement of airflow limitation by fluticasone propionate/salmeterol in chronic obstructive pulmonary disease: what is the specific marker? Front Pharmacol. 2011;2:36. https://doi.org/10.3389/fphar.2011.00036.
17. Christenson SA, Steiling K, van den Berge M, Hijazi K, Hiemstra PS, Postma DS, Lenburg ME, Spira A, Woodruff PG. Asthma-COPD overlap. Clinical relevance of genomic signatures of type 2 inflammation in chronic obstructive pulmonary disease. Am J Respir Crit Care Med. 2015;191:758–66.

Chapter 10
Aspirin-Exacerbated Respiratory Disease (AERD)

Masami Taniguchi, Chihiro Mitsui, and Hiroaki Hayashi

Abstract The characteristics in AERD are severe asthma, eosinophilic rhinosinusitis, and cysteinyl leukotriene (CysLT) overproduction. The interaction between platelets and granulocytes leads to the CysLT overproduction and severe eosinophilic inflammation. The ongoing activation of mast cells is key pathogenesis in not only stable AERD but exacerbated AERD by aspirin. Omalizumab is an effective option for AERD via suppression of mast cell activation.

Keywords AERD · Leukotriene · Severe asthma · Omalizumab · Eosinophilic sinusitis

10.1 Introduction and Definition

Aspirin-exacerbated respiratory disease (AERD) is caused not by an allergic reaction to aspirin but by a non-allergic hypersensitivity (intolerance) that produces severe respiratory symptoms (congested nose, nasal discharge, and asthma attacks) caused by nonsteroidal anti-inflammatory drugs (NSAIDs), such as aspirin, that inhibit cyclooxygenase (COX), a synthetic enzyme of prostaglandins (PGs) [1–3]. A hypersensitivity reaction in AERD is more frequently induced by NSAIDs that have a stronger COX-1 inhibitory activity. In contrast, a selective COX-2 inhibitor, such as celecoxib, can be safely used in patients with AERD [3–5]. From these findings, it is concluded that the hypersensitivity reaction in AERD is caused by a COX-1 inhibition [1–5].

M. Taniguchi (✉) · C. Mitsui · H. Hayashi
Clinical Research Center, Sagamihara National Hospital, Sagamihara, Kanagawa, Japan
e-mail: m-taniguchi@sagamihara-hosp.gr.jp

A. Yokoyama (ed.), *Advances in Asthma*, Respiratory Disease Series: Diagnostic Tools and Disease Managements, https://doi.org/10.1007/978-981-13-2790-2_10

10.2 Epidemiological and Clinical Findings

AERD is rare among children. The frequency of AERD is ~5–10% of patients with adult-onset asthma [2, 3, 6, 7], and the ratio of male and female patients is 1:2 [6]. Usual patients with AERD have a severe asthma; therefore, the percentage of patients with AERD among asthma is high at specialist hospital, whereas it is less than 5% at general clinics [7]. According to a European-wide study, the average age of AERD onset is 35 years, and according to studies in the USA and Japan, it is 36 years. Namely, people in their 20s–40s tend to develop AERD. Familial AERD has been reported in 1–2% of patients with AERD. Differences in the percentage of patients with AERD among races and regions have not been reported. The typical clinical features of AERD are as follows. The type of asthma in AERD is a nonatopic or weakly atopic constitution, and their almost all asthma onset in AERD is after adolescence [8]. Patients with severe asthma account for more than half of patients with AERD [8]. They tend to develop a persistent airflow obstruction after the inhalation of a β2 agonist [9]. As explained, AERD is a typical intractable adult-onset asthma [10, 11]. In particular, nonatopic asthma in female patients with AERD tends to become intractable [12]. However, there are some (~10%) patients whose symptoms are mild and such patients only develop asthma attacks when they take NSAIDs. The mechanisms of intractable AERD have remained unclear [1–3].

A severe nasal obstruction, nasal discharge, and asthma exacerbation are induced by usual dose of NSAIDs in patients with AERD. They often show facial flushing and conjunctival reddening derived from histamine overproduction. GI symptoms (abdominal pain, nausea, and diarrhea), chest pain, itching, and urticaria are sometimes observed in a third of patients with AERD. The hypersensitivity reaction in AERD appears within 1 h from ingestion of NSAIDs. The appearance of NSAID-hypersensitivity symptom is sometimes delayed when slow-releasing tablets or transdermal patches are used.

The most important characteristic of clinical feature in AERD is eosinophilic rhinosinusitis with nasal polyposis that may lead to hyposmia [2]. More than half of adult patients with moderate-severe asthma who have nasal polyposis complicated with AERD. Nasal symptoms (particularly hyposmia) generally develop several years before the onset of AERD. Currently, the symptoms of asthma are often stabilized by inhaled corticosteroid (=ICS) therapy; however, symptoms other than those in the lower respiratory tract become noticeable [2]. In recent years, eosinophilic otitis media, eosinophilic enteritis, and variant angina-like chest pain have been observed in more than half, ~30%, and 10–20% of patients with AERD, respectively [2]. Peripheral blood eosinophilia is more prominent in patients with moderate-severe AERD than in those with aspirin-tolerant asthma (ATA).

Ten to 20% of patients with AERD show a hypersensitivity reaction (mainly, coughing) to several kinds of mint and toothpaste containing them [2]. The mechanism for this is unclear; however, it is considered that the chemical structure of mint is similar to that of salicylates. It was previously reported that patients with AERD show a hypersensitivity reaction to colorings (such as tartrazine), additives, and natural salicylates contained in fruits and vegetables. However, the symptoms of asthma do not significantly worsen when patients orally ingest them in typical amounts, and the proof of the benefit of avoiding them is insufficient [13]. Note that the prompt administration of drugs (inhalation drugs [14] and liquid drugs) containing additives (particularly, parabens and metabisulfate) may induce a hypersensitivity reaction in patients with unstable AERD. Some spices contain high contents of natural salicylates, the intake of which may worsen symptoms in patients with AERD.

10.3 Causes and Pathogenetic Mechanism of AERD

Familial AERD is rare, and no strong genetic basis has been observed. There is no relationship between the past history of NSAID administration and the onset of AERD. As the pathogenic mechanism, autoimmune mechanism, chronic viral infection, and an allergic reaction to the superantigen of *Staphylococcus aureus* have been considered. However, none of them are based on substantial grounds. The reasons why AERD is acquired (not congenital) or easily has the complication of eosinophilic rhinosinusitis have remained unclarified.

10.4 Typical Pathological Conditions

There are three typical pathological conditions of AERD: (1) severe asthma, (2) eosinophilic rhinosinusitis, and (3) cysteinyl leukotriene (CysLT) hyperproduction [15–18].

The urinary concentration of leukotriene E_4 (LTE_4), a stable metabolic product of cysteinyl leukotriene (Cyst), is three- to fivefold higher in patients with stable AERD than in patients with stable ATA (Fig. 10.1a). The urinary LTE4 concentration significantly decreases after an endoscopic nasal surgery of nasal polyposis (Fig. 10.1b). The urinary LTE_4 concentration increases 2–30-fold during aspirin provocation test [15–18]. Other typical pathological conditions are an imbalance of eicosanoids and decreases in the production of the anti-inflammatory mediator, prostaglandin E_2 (PGE_2) [18] and lipoxin (Fig. 10.2) [19]. The decrease in the production of PGE_2 caused by the reduction in COX-2 activity [20], especially the attenuation of PGE_2 receptor subtype 2 (EP2) stimulation, is considered to be related to the three abovementioned typical pathological conditions of AERD. However, there have been no animal models of AERD, and in vitro-specific reactions have not been confirmed thus far. The reason for the acquired (not congenital) imbalance of eicosanoids has not been clarified [1–3]. In addition, the following are still unknown:

(1) whether the imbalance of eicosanoids (Fig. 10.2) is observed throughout the body or only in the respiratory tract, (2) which cells show a hypersensitivity reaction to COX-1 inhibitors, and (3) why patients show a hypersensitivity reaction to even a small amount of aspirin.

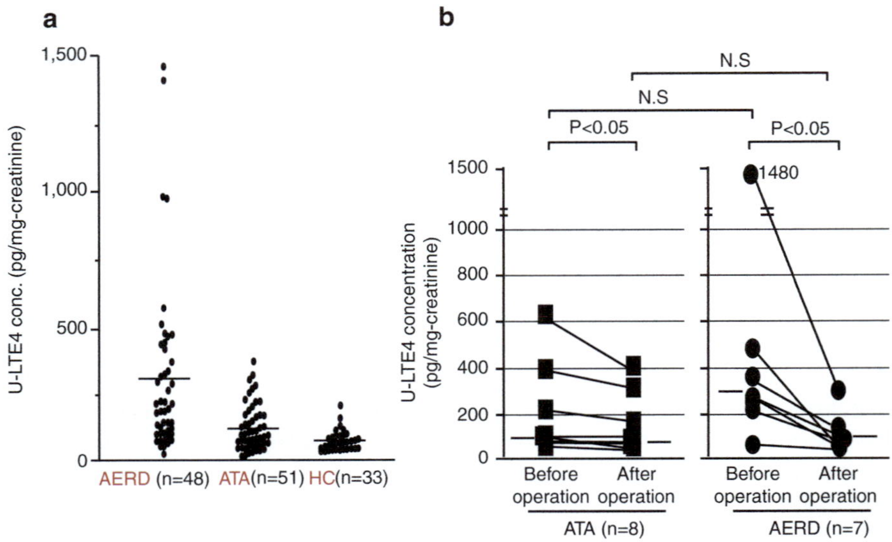

Fig. 10.1 (**a**) The urinary LTE4 concentration in patients with AERD and ATA during stable condition. (**b**) The urinary LTE4 concentration decreases significantly after the operation to remove nasal polyps. The concentration in some patients falls within the normal range

Fig. 10.2 Imbalance of arachidonic acid metabolites in patients with AERD (hypothesis). The COX-2 level decreases in patients with AERD and the production of endogenous PGE2 also decreases. With the addition of a COX-1 inhibitor, the amount of PGE2 further decreases, the suppression of 5-lipoxygenase (5-LO) activity disappears, and CysLT is overproduced

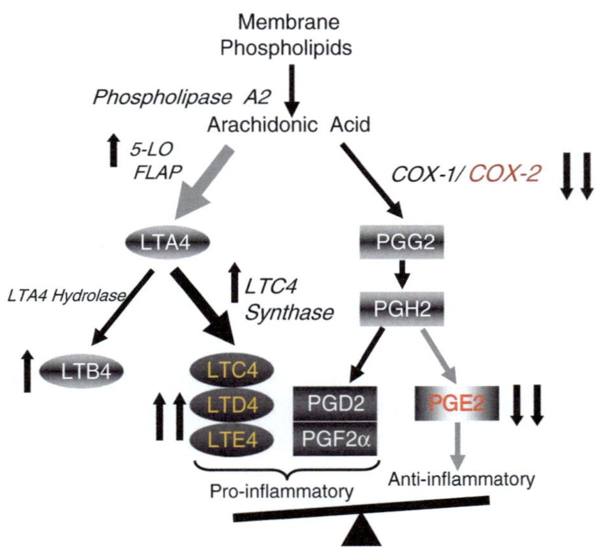

10.5 Involvement of Platelets

Platelets are crucially involved in the development of allergic diseases, including bronchial asthma. Platelets in asthmatics are more activated than those in healthy individuals. Platelets are considered to be involved in the development of AERD because (1) AERD is induced after the administration of ≤100 mg of aspirin (a small amount of aspirin that mainly inhibits COX-1 in platelets), (2) there is a refractory period of 3–7 days after the administration of aspirin [21] (this refractory period is specific to AERD and almost corresponds to the lifetime of platelets), and (3) patients with AERD are sensitive to COX-1 inhibitors but tolerant to COX-2 inhibitors (among the cells in the human body, only platelets contain COX-1 alone). The group of Laidlaw and Boyce [22] and Mitsui et al. [23] reported the specific activation of platelets as well as the frequent adhesion with granulocytes and platelets in peripheral blood and the respiratory tract of patients with AERD. Their findings correspond reasonably well to our hypothesis. These phenomena are not observed in patients with severe ATA or chronic eosinophilic pneumonia [23]. The activated platelets and adhesion molecules, such as P selectin, lead to the adhesion of platelets and inflammatory granulocytes or respiratory epithelium. The interaction between platelets and granulocytes is considered to lead to the overproduction of CysLT and severe eosinophilic inflammation (Fig. 10.3) [23]. However, no significant change in the platelet activation marker is observed during aspirin provocation test [23]. Very recently, Laidlaw et al. reported that P2Y12 receptor antagonist (prasugrel) did not attenuate AERD symptoms [24].

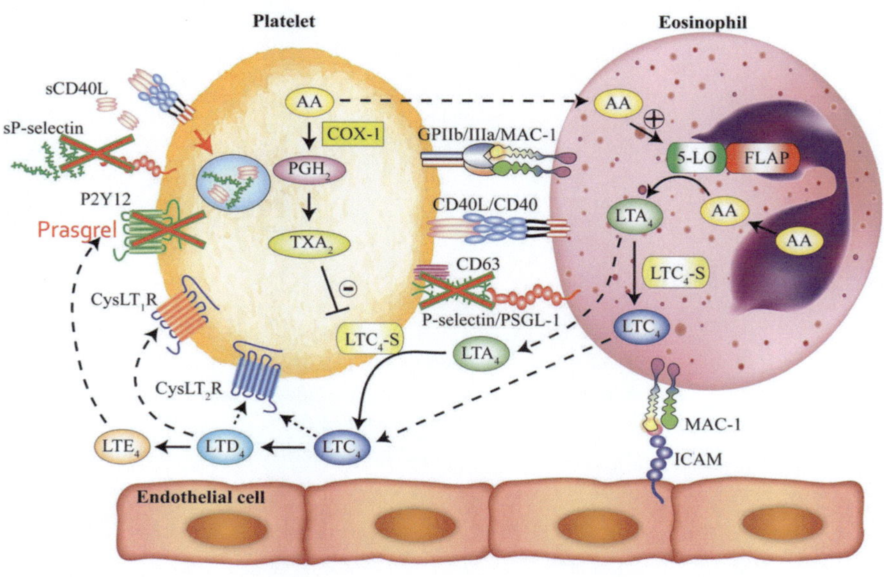

Fig. 10.3 New hypothesis of AERD development. Is the cross talk between platelets and granulocytes the cause of AERD?

10.6 Role of Mast Cells

During aspirin reactions, many mediators are released including CysLT, tryptase, histamine, and prostaglandin D2 (PGD2) suggesting mast cell activation [25–28]. Concentration of PGD2 level, which is a marker of mast cell activation, is significantly high in their sputum, blood, and exhaled breath condensate in patients with stable AERD, even in those using ICS [28]. Single bronchial inhalation of sodium cromoglycate (a mast cell stabilizer) rapidly improves their pulmonary functions especially in patients with stable AERD (Fig. 10.4) [29]. On the basis of these findings, the ongoing activation of mast cells is one of the characteristics of pathogenesis in not only stable AERD but also exacerbated AERD by aspirin.

During oral aspirin challenge test, urinary level of PGD2M (=mast cell activation marker) levels significantly increases. Because there is a positive correlation between the urinary LTE4 concentration and PGD2M concentration, the aspirin-induced hypersensitive reactions are mainly caused by mast cells. Both aspirin-induced reaction and acute allergic reaction (anaphylaxis) via immunoglobulin E (IgE) might be similar mechanism. However, in the case of IgE-anaphylaxis, PGD2 is dominant, whereas CysLT is dominant in aspirin-induced reaction with AERD. The precise mechanism underlying the mutual activation of mast cells has not yet been clarified.

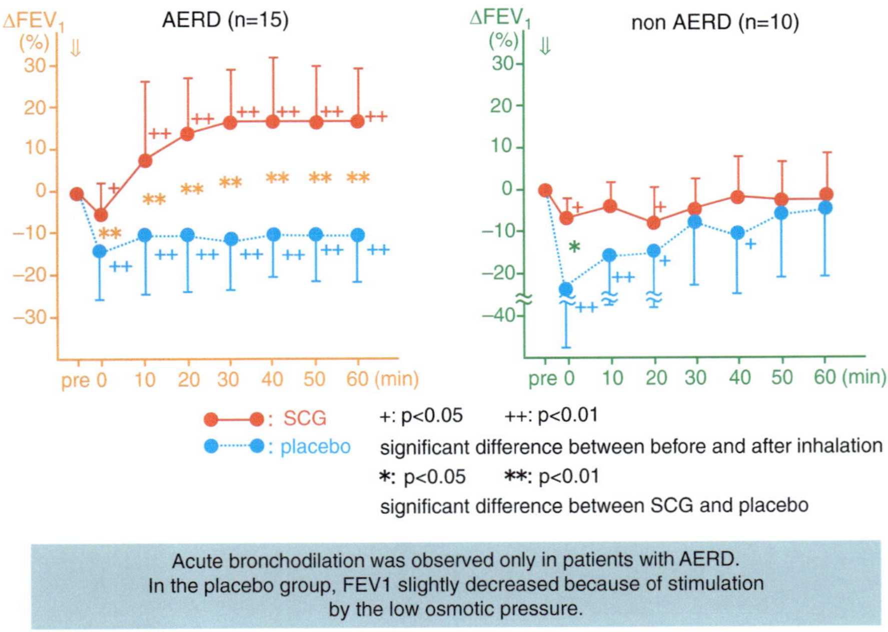

Fig. 10.4 Change in FEV1 in patients with AERD who inhaled Intal® (SCG) and a placebo group (patients who inhaled saline solution with the same osmotic pressure as that of SCG)

10.7 Involvement of Basophils and Innate Lymphoid Type 2 Cells (ILC2)

Although the main CysLT-producing cells are mast cells and basophils in human, basophils are not activated in the peripheral blood in patients with AERD in stable condition and during an aspirin challenge test [30]. In recent years, eosinophilic nasal polyps and type 2 inflammation caused by ILC2 activation in patients with AERD have been attracting attention [31, 32]. The involvement of ILC2 in the induction of AERD is expected because the pathological conditions caused by an increase in the number of eosinophils, rather than stimulation by an allergen, are the main symptoms.

10.8 Common Pathological Conditions of Eosinophilic Nasal Polyp and AERD: Decrease in COX-2 Level (Fig. 10.5)

Figure 10.5 shows the relationship among the number of inflammatory cells and the levels of cytokine, chemokine, and various mediators in patients with chronic rhinosinusitis (CRS in Fig. 10.5), chronic rhinosinusitis with a nasal polyp (CRS + NP), and chronic rhinosinusitis with AERD complicated with a nasal polyp (CRS + NP + AERD). This figure summarizes the findings of previous reports. Patients with AERD

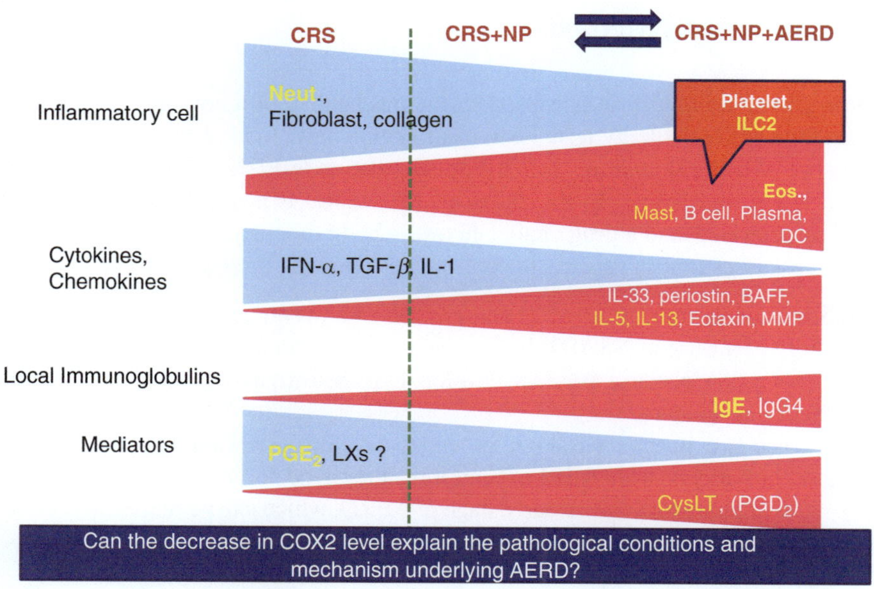

Fig. 10.5 Are CRS + NP and CRS + NP + AERD continuous pathological conditions? This figure shows a summary of the findings of past reports and our experience)

have more severe pathological conditions than CRS + NP. It is considered that the pathomechanisms of AERD and eosinophilic nasal polyps are quantitatively different but qualitatively the same. This is consistent with the clinical findings for patients with AERD and those with ATA and a nasal polyp. The basic idea that can explain all the above phenomena is considered to be the decrease in COX level. On the basis of the results of analysis of COX activity in knockout mice [33–36] and histopathological analysis of nasal polyps [37, 38], a decrease in COX-2 level can consistently explain the three typical pathological conditions of patients with AERD and eosinophilic rhinosinusitis described in Sect. 10.4 [39, 40]. Furthermore, the underlying mechanism is considered to be the attenuation in the EP2 receptor function (anti-inflammatory function) caused by the impaired production of endogenous PGE2 owing to the decrease in COX-2 level. The research group of Boyce demonstrated that PGE2-1-synthesis-enzyme-deficient mice show pathological conditions similar to those of AERD and that the inflammatory symptoms can be improved by treatment with an EP2 receptor agonist [33]. However, insufficient proof has been obtained thus far. In addition, the cells and tissues in which a decrease in COX-2 level has a significant effect have not yet identified, and the reason for the acquisition of AERD (not congenital) has not yet been determined. Hayashi et al. have recently reported the possibility that smoking, which induces COX-2 in the respiratory tract, inhibits the onset of AERD in humans, because people who quit smoking tend to develop asthma within 5 years of quitting and, among patients who smoke, the number of AERD patients is statistically significantly smaller than that of ATA patients [41].

10.9 Diagnosis Method

Hypersensitivity to aspirin is caused by the mechanism of a non-allergic reaction. Therefore, general allergy tests (skin examination and blood tests) are not used to diagnose AERD [3]. A drug lymphocyte stimulation test (DLST) using peripheral blood is also not helpful in the diagnosis [3]. AERD is basically diagnosed by a medical interview and a drug challenge test [42]. In the medical interview, doctors should ask questions to patients to confirm the following three points:

1. History of the use of NSAIDs and any adverse events related to their use: the history of the use of NSAIDs before the onset of asthma should not be taken into consideration because patients develop hypersensitivity to NSAIDs after the onset of asthma.
2. Presence of hyposmia: nasal polyps tend to develop in the vicinity of the ethmoid sinus in patients with AERD. Therefore, they tend to complain of hyposmia (~90% of patients) from an early stage of AERD, which can be transiently recovered by the administration of systemic steroids.
3. Histories of nasal polyps and rhinosinusitis and surgical history.

In addition, if a patient satisfies two or more items from among the following clinical backgrounds, in addition to the above three items, the patient is strongly suspected of having AERD. The clinical backgrounds include moderate or severe asthma, the onset of asthma after adolescence, a weakly atopic disposition, asthma with an intractable cough, and ≥10% increase in peripheral eosinophilia.

The gold standard for making a definitive diagnosis is the aspirin oral challenge test [3]. It is desirable to carry out the test at a specialized institution with experienced doctors when the symptoms of the patient are in a stable period. The details of the aspirin challenge test are given in [3, 42].

10.10 Specific Therapies

(1) We have pointed out in our previous reports that the rapid intravenous injection of steroids may cause a severe asthma attack [28–30]. The chemical structure of steroids and endogenous steroids is insoluble in water. The steroids used for intravenous injection have the ester structure of phosphoric acid or succinic acid. Patients with AERD show a hypersensitivity reaction to the chemical structure of succinic acid steroids. Therefore, the rapid intravenous injection of succinate ester steroids should be avoided for patients with AERD. Also, the rapid intravenous injection of other types of steroids with several additives should therefore be avoided. Intravenous drip injection over at least 1–2 h is recommended [2, 43].

(2) It was demonstrated that cromolyn (Intal®), a mast cell stabilizer, is an effective candidate for patients with unstable AERD [29]. The mechanism behind this is considered to be the continuous activation of mast cells in the respiratory tract of patients with AERD.

(3) Hayashi et al. reported that omalizumab is very effective for AERD and acts rapidly [44]. They also reported that the mechanism behind this is the suppression of mast cell activation (production of PGD2) and CysLT overproduction (Fig. 10.6) rather than the suppression of eosinophilic inflammation [44]. Omalizumab suppresses mast cell activation in patients with intractable urticaria and is rapidly effective. It is also considered that omalizumab is effective as a mast cell stabilizer for patients with AERD. The current approach to treating intractable AERD is the use of omalizumab in addition to the drugs that the patient generally takes. For patients with severe eosinophilic inflammation, the combined use of omalizumab with interleukin (IL)-5 is also an option.

(4) Adrenaline is effective for all types of NSAID-induced acute symptoms of patients with AERD [2]. This is because the pathological conditions, such as systemic vascular leakage, induced and the increased production of mediators are similar to the anaphylactic reactions via IgE [18, 27].

	Characteristic pathological condition (AERD vs ATA)	Severe pathological condition (severe vs nonsevere AERD)	Mechanism of omalizumab action (ref:44)
Aspirin-hypersensitivity	◎	→	? ? ?
Severe asthma	◎	↑ ↑	↓
Nasal polyposis	◎	↑	↓
Cys-LT overproduction (unpublished data)	◎	↑ ↑	↓ ↓
Severe eos.inflammation	○	↑	↓
Mast cell activation (ref: 25-29)	○	↑	↓ ↓
Platelet activation (ref: 23,24)	○	?	?
Neutrophil activation (unpublished data)	—	↗	?
Basophil activation (ref: 30)	—	→	?

Fig. 10.6 Characteristic and severe pathological conditions of AERD and mechanism of omalizumab action

10.11 Conclusion

The specific pathomechanism of AERD is not only mast cell activation but platelet and ILC2 activation. Recent reports claim that anti-IgE treatment is a strong candidate for intractable AERD patients via mast cell stabilization. In the future, antiplatelet and anti-ILC2 drugs may be a useful option for AERD.

References

1. Stevenson DD, Szczeklik A. Clinical and pathologic perspectives on aspirin sensitivity and asthma. J Allergy Clin Immunol. 2006;118:773–86.
2. Taniguchi M. Aspirin-exacerbated respiratory disease (AERD). Nippon Naika Gakkai Zasshi. 2013;102(6):1426–32.
3. Kowalski ML, Makowska JS, Blanca M, et al. Hypersensitivity to nonsteroidal anti-inflammatory drugs (NSAIDs) -classification, diagnosis and management: review of the EAACI/ENDA(#) and GA2LEN/HANNA. Allergy. 2011;66:818–29.
4. Szczeklik A, Sanak M. The role of COX-1 and COX-2 in asthma pathogenesis and its significance in the use of selective inhibitors. Clin Exp Allergy. 2002;32:339–42.
5. Morales DR, Lipworth BJ, Guthrie B, et al. Safety risks for patients with aspirin-exacerbated respiratory disease after acute exposure to selective nonsteroidal anti-inflammatory drugs and COX-2 inhibitors: Meta-analysis of controlled clinical trials. J Allergy Clin Immunol. 2014;134(1):40–5.

6. Fukutomi Y, Taniguchi M, Tsuburai T, Okada C, Shimoda T, Onaka A, Saka H, Sadakane A, Nakamura K, Akiyama K, National Hospital Organization Research Network for Asthma. Survey of asthma control and anti-asthma medication use among Japanese adult patients. Arerugi. 2010;59(1):37–46.
7. Rajan JP, Wineinger NE, Stevenson DD, White AA. Prevalence of aspirin-exacerbated respiratory disease among asthmatic patients: a meta-analysis of the literature. J Allergy Clin Immunol. 2014;135(3):676–81.
8. Szczeklik A, Nizankowska E, Duplaga M. Natural history of aspirin-induced asthma. AIANE Investigators. European network on aspirin-induced asthma. Eur Respir J. 2000;16:432–6.
9. Mascia K, Haselkorn T, Deniz YM, et al. Aspirin sensitivity and severity of asthma: evidence for irreversible airway obstruction in patients with severe or difficult-to-treat asthma. J Allergy Clin Immunol. 2005;116:970–5.
10. Group TES. The ENFUMOSA cross-sectional European multicentre study of the clinical phenotype of chronic severe asthma. European network for understanding mechanisms of severe asthma. Eur Respir J. 2003;22:470–7.
11. Moore WC, Bleecker ER, Curran-Everett D, et al. Characterization of the severe asthma phenotype by the National Heart, Lung, and Blood Institute's Severe Asthma Research Program. J Allergy Clin Immunol. 2007;119:405–13.
12. Fukutomi Y, Taniguchi M, Tsuburai T, et al. Obesity and aspirin intolerance are risk factors for difficult-to-treat asthma in Japanese non-atopic women. Clin Exp Allergy. 2012;42:738–46.
13. Virchow C, Szczeklik A, Bianco S, et al. Intolerance to tartrazine in aspirin-induced asthma: results of a multicenter study. Respiration. 1988;53:20–3.
14. Abo M, Fujimura M. Tacholiquine inhalation and aspirin-induced asthma. Chest. 2001;119:670.
15. Christie PE, Tagari P, Ford-Hutchinson AW, et al. Urinary leukotriene E4 concentrations increase after aspirin challenge in aspirin-sensitive asthmatic subjects. Am Rev Respir Dis. 1991;143(5 Pt1):1025–9.
16. Kawagishi Y, Mita H, Taniguchi M, et al. Leukotriene C4 synthase promoter polymorphism in Japanese patients with aspirin-induced asthma. J Allergy Clin Immunol. 2002;109:936–42.
17. Higashi N, Taniguchi M, Mita H, et al. Clinical features of asthmatic patients with increased urinary leukotriene E4 excretion (hyperleukotrienuria):Involvement of chronic hyperplastic rhinosinusitis with nasal polyposis. J Allergy Clin Immunol. 2004;113:277–83.
18. Higashi N, Mita H, Ono E, et al. Profile of eicosanoid generation in aspirin-intolerant asthma and anaphylaxis assessed by new biomarkers. J Allergy Clin Immunol. 2010;125:1084–91.
19. Yamaguchi H, Higashi N, Mita H, et al. Urinary concentrations of 15-epimer of lipoxin A(4) are lower in patients with aspirin-intolerant compared with aspirin-tolerant asthma. Clin Exp Allergy. 2011;41:1711–8.
20. Picado C, Fernandez-Morata JC, Juan M, et al. Cyclooxygenase-2 mRNA is downexpressed in nasal polyps from aspirin-sensitive asthmatics. Am J Respir Crit Care Med. 1999;160:291–6.
21. Pleskow WW, Stevenson DD, Mathison DA, Simon RA, Schatz M, Zeiger RS. Aspirin desensitization in aspirin-sensitive asthmatic patients: clinical manifestations and characterization of the refractory period. J Allergy Clin Immunol. 1982;69(1 Pt 1):11–9.
22. Laidlaw TM, Kidder MS, Bhattacharyya N, Xing W, Shen S, Milne GL, Castells MC, Chhay H, Boyce JA. Cysteinyl leukotriene overproduction in aspirin-exacerbated respiratory disease is driven by platelet-adherent leukocytes. Blood. 2012;119(16):3790–8.
23. Mitsui C, Kajiwara K, Hayashi H, et al. Platelet activation markers overexpressed specifically in patients with aspirin-exacerbated respiratory disease. J Allergy Clin Immunol. 2016;137(2):400–11.
24. Laidlaw TM, Cahill KN, Cardet JC, Murphy K, Cui J, Dioneda B, Kothari P, Raby BA, Israel E, Boyce JA. A trial of type 12 purinergic (P2Y(12)) receptor inhibition with prasugrel identifies a potentially distinct endotype of patients with aspirin-exacerbated respiratory disease. J Allergy Clin Immunol. 2018. https://doi.org/10.1016/j.jaci.2018.06.001

25. Mita H, Endoh S, Kudoh M, Kawagishi Y, Kobayashi M, Taniguchi M, Akiyama K. Possible involvement of mast-cell activation in aspirin provocation of aspirin-induced asthma. Allergy. 2001;56(11):1061–7.
26. Higashi N, Taniguchi M, Mita H, Yamaguchi H, Ono E, Akiyama K. Aspirin-intolerant asthma (AIA) assessment using the urinary biomarkers, leukotriene E4 (LTE4) and prostaglandin D2 (PGD2) metabolites. Allergol Int. 2012;61(3):393–403.
27. Higashi N, Mita H, Yamaguchi H, Fukutomi Y, Akiyama K, Taniguchi M. Urinary tetranor-PGDM concentrations in aspirin-intolerant asthma and anaphylaxis. J Allergy Clin Immunol. 2012;129(2):557–9.
28. Higashi N, Taniguchi M, Mita H, Osame M, Akiyama K. A comparative study of eicosanoid concentrations in sputum and urine in patients with aspirin-intolerant asthma. Clin Exp Allergy. 2002;32(10):1484–90.
29. Imokawa S, Sato A, Taniguchi M, Toyoshima M, Nakazawa K, Hayakawa H, Chida K. Sodium cromoglycate nebulized solution has an acute bronchodilative effect in patients with aspirin-intolerant asthma (AIA). Arerugi. 1992;41(10):1515–20.
30. Mitsui C, Kajiwara K, Ono E, Watai K, Hayashi H, Kamide Y, Fukutomi Y, Sekiya K, Tsuburai T, Yamamoto K, Taniguchi M. Analysis of basophil activation in patients with aspirin-exacerbated respiratory disease. J Allergy Clin Immunol. 2017;140(4):1162–4.
31. White AA, Doherty TA. Role of group 2 innate lymphocytes in aspirin-exacerbated respiratory disease pathogenesis. Am J Rhinol Allergy. 2018;32(1):7–11.
32. Liu T, Barrett NA, Kanaoka Y, Yoshimoto E, Garofalo D, Cirka H, Feng C, Boyce JA. Type 2 cysteinyl leukotriene receptors drive IL-33-dependent type 2 immunopathology and aspirin sensitivity. J Immunol. 2018;200(3):915–27.
33. Liu T, Laidlaw TM, Katz HR, Boyce JA. Prostaglandin E2 deficiency causes a phenotype of aspirin sensitivity that depends on platelets and cysteinyl leukotrienes. Proc Natl Acad Sci U S A. 2013;110(42):16987–92.
34. Li H, Bradbury JA, Dackor RT, Edin ML, Graves JP, DeGraff LM, Wang PM, Bortner CD, Maruoka S, Lih FB, Cook DN, Tomer KB, Jetten AM, Zeldin DC. Cyclooxygenase-2 regulates Th17 cell differentiation during allergic lung inflammation. Am J Respir Crit Care Med. 2011;184(1):37–49.
35. Harrington LS, Lucas R, McMaster SK, Moreno L, Scadding G, Warner TD, Mitchell JA. COX-1, and not COX-2 activity, regulates airway function: relevance to aspirin-sensitive asthma. FASEB J. 2008;22(11):4005–10.
36. Nakata J, Kondo M, Tamaoki J, Takemiya T, Nohara M, Yamagata K, Nagai A. Augmentation of allergic inflammation in the airways of cyclooxygenase-2-deficient mice. Respirology. 2005;10(2):149–56.
37. Pezato R, Świerczyńska-Krępa M, Niżankowska-Mogilnicka E, Holtappels G, De Ruyck N, Sanak M, Derycke L, Van Crombruggen K, Bachert C, Pérez-Novo CA. Systemic expression of inflammatory mediators in patients with chronic rhinosinusitis and nasal polyps with and without Aspirin Exacerbated Respiratory Disease. Cytokine. 2016;77:157–67.
38. Pérez-Novo CA, Kowalski ML, Kuna P, Ptasinska A, Holtappels G, van Cauwenberge P, Gevaert P, Johannson S, Bachert C. Aspirin sensitivity and IgE antibodies to Staphylococcus aureus enterotoxins in nasal polyposis: studies on the relationship. Int Arch Allergy Immunol. 2004;133(3):255–60.
39. Ying S, Meng Q, Scadding G, Parikh A, Corrigan CJ, Lee TH. Aspirin-sensitive rhinosinusitis is associated with reduced E-prostanoid 2 receptor expression on nasal mucosal inflammatory cells. J Allergy Clin Immunol. 2006;117(2):312–8.
40. Roca-Ferrer J, Garcia-Garcia FJ, Pereda J, Perez-Gonzalez M, Pujols L, Alobid I, Mullol J, Picado C. Reduced expression of COXs and production of prostaglandin E(2) in patients with nasal polyps with or without aspirin-intolerant asthma. J Allergy Clin Immunol. 2011;128(1):66–72.
41. Hayashi H, Fukutomi Y, Mitsui C, Nakatani E, Watai K, Kamide Y, Sekiya K, Tsuburai T, Ito S, Hasegawa Y, Taniguchi M. Smoking cessation as a possible risk factor for the develop-

ment of aspirin-exacerbated respiratory disease in smokers. J Allergy Clin Immunol Pract. 2018;6(1):116–125.e3.
42. Taniguchi M. Measurement of airway hyperresponsiveness and aspirin sensitivity. Arerugi. 2009;58(2):87–96.
43. Szczeklik A. Hypersensitivity to systemic corticosteroids in aspirin-sensitive patients with asthma. J Allergy Clin Immunol. 2011;128:904–5.
44. Hayashi H, Mitsui C, Nakatani E, Fukutomi Y, Kajiwara K, Watai K, Sekiya K, Tsuburai T, Akiyama K, Hasegawa Y, Taniguchi M. Omalizumab reduces cysteinyl leukotriene and 9α,11β-prostaglandin F2 overproduction in aspirin-exacerbated respiratory disease. J Allergy Clin Immunol. 2016;137(5):1585–7.

Part III
Treatment

Chapter 11
Essence of the Japanese Guidelines for Adult Asthma

Tomohiro Ichikawa and Hisatoshi Sugiura

Abstract The Japanese guidelines for adult asthma were first published in 1993 and have been updated every 3 years. The latest version of Japanese guidelines was updated in 2015 and the English version was published in 2017 (JGL 2017). In the latest guidelines, the definition, management, and treatment of asthma have been modified. In this chapter, we described the contents of the Japanese guidelines as compared to the Global Initiative for Asthma (GINA) guidelines, especially focusing on treatment. In the JGL, the initial treatment and long-term management of asthma have been based on a stepwise approach. In the JGL, determination of the treatment steps differs between untreated and treated patients. In stable asthma, the use of low dose inhaled corticosteroid is recommended for the initial treatment at step 1 treatment in JGL because the goal of asthma management in JGL is to eliminate the symptoms. In contrast, no controller drug is recommended as the basic treatment at the step 1 treatment in GINA. This chapter overviews the treatment plans for asthma management in the Japanese guidelines and discusses some differences in the approach from GINA.

Keywords Japanese guidelines for adult asthma · Goal of asthma treatment · Stepwise approach

---

T. Ichikawa (✉) · H. Sugiura
Department of Respiratory Medicine, Tohoku University Graduate School of Medicine, Sendai, Japan
e-mail: ichikawa@rm.med.tohoku.ac.jp

A. Yokoyama (ed.), *Advances in Asthma*, Respiratory Disease Series: Diagnostic Tools and Disease Managements, https://doi.org/10.1007/978-981-13-2790-2_11

11.1 Introduction

The Japanese guidelines for adult asthma, termed "Asthma Prevention and Management Guidelines" (JGL) were first published in 1993 and have been updated every three years. JGL 2015, the last updated version of Japanese guideline, has been published and the English version of JGL 2015, "Japanese guidelines for adult asthma 2017" [1] is now available. In the JGL, the treatment steps for long-term management are determined based on the severity in untreated patients. In patients under treatment, the treatment steps are determined by the current treatment steps and asthma symptoms. "No asthma related symptoms" is set as the ideal goal of asthma management in the JGL. This chapter introduces asthma medications for the long-term management and for asthma exacerbations in the JGL, and discusses the key differences from the Global Initiative for Asthma (GINA) [2], the global guidelines for asthma management and prevention.

11.2 Definition of Asthma and Aims of Asthma Management

Adult bronchial asthma is defined as a disease that is characterized by chronic airway inflammation, clinically presenting variable airway narrowing (wheezes and dyspnea) and cough [1], and especially variability is highlighted in the definition, similar to the GINA. Airway narrowing is reversible and derives from airway inflammation and airway hyperresponsiveness. In these respects, the aim of asthma management and treatment is to achieve an improvement of the airway hyperresponsiveness and airflow limitation by eliminating inducers of airway inflammation, by adopting pharmacotherapy to alleviate inflammation, and by dilating the constricted airway [1]. The clinical diagnosis of asthma is based on the key features of asthma [3–6]. The definition, aims, and diagnosis appear to be similar to those in GINA.

11.3 Long-Term Management of Asthma

11.3.1 Principle for Treatment

The goal of asthma treatment is to achieve normal respiratory function, with an absence of symptoms, exacerbations, or adverse effects. Asthma control is assessed according to Table 11.1 with the aim being to achieve a "Well controlled" status. The differences of definition of asthma control status between in JGL and in GINA are also shown in Table 11.1.

Furthermore, the aim of drug therapy is to achieve the maximum effect using the minimum number or dosage of asthma drugs. For these purposes, a stepwise

Table 11.1 Assessment of asthma control in Japanese guidelines (JGL) and GINA

Assessment items		JGL	GINA
Asthma symptoms	Daytime	More than once a week	More than twice a week
	At night		Any
Use of reliever		More than once a week	More than twice a week
Limitation of activities		Any	Any
Lung function (FEV1 and PEF)		Predicted value or ≥80% of the best value	Not included (listed in risk factors for exacerbation)
Diurnal (weekly) variation in PEF		≥20%	Not included
Exacerbations		More than once a year[a]/once a month[b]	Not included

Definition of asthma control status in JGL and GINA is as follows: *JGL* well-controlled if patients meet no criteria listed in the table; insufficient if patients have at least one or two criteria; poorly-controlled if patients have more than three criteria, *GINA* well-controlled if patients meet no criteria listed in the table; partly controlled if patients have one or two criteria; uncontrolled if patients have three or four of the criteria

[a]Criteria for insufficient control

[b]Define patients with one or more exacerbations a month as being poorly controlled, even if they do not meet the other criteria

approach is applied for asthma management in JGL. JGL divides asthma treatments into 4 treatment steps (Table 11.2).

Treatment steps are determined based on the severity of asthma in untreated patients (Table 11.3). In the patients under treatment, the treatment steps are determined by the current treatment steps and asthma symptoms (Table 11.4). The details of the stepwise approach using these categorizations are described in another section.

11.3.2 Medications and Treatment Options

Asthma medications are divided into two categories, controllers and relievers. Controllers are drugs that are used continuously for long-term management to achieve good control of asthma including inhaled corticosteroid (ICS), long-acting β2 agonists (LABA), leukotriene receptor antagonists (LTRA), sustained release theophylline and long-acting muscarinic antagonists (LAMA). Anti-IgE antibody (omalizumab) and anti-IL-5 antibody (mepolizumab) are also categorized as controllers. Relievers are drugs used for short term to treat asthma exacerbations such as short-acting β2 agonists (SABA) and oral corticosteroid (OCS). In contrast to GINA, immunosuppressive agents such as cyclosporine and methotrexate, and gold are not recommended in the JGL because evidence for these agents is insufficient. Tulobuterol patch, an adhesive transdermal patch containing a β2-agonist and developed in Japan, is described as a LABA only in the JGL. It is useful for patients in whom inhalation and oral administration are difficult. The clinical usefulness when

Table 11.2 Treatment steps of Japanese guidelines and GINA

Japanese guidelines for both untreated patients and long-term management					
		Treatment step 1	**Treatment step 2**	**Treatment step 3**	**Treatment step 4**
Long-term management agents	Basic treatment	Low dose ICS	Low to medium doses ICS	Medium to high doses ICS	High dose ICS
		If the above agent cannot be used, use one of the following agents • LTRA • Theophylline sustained-release preparation (unnecessary for rare symptoms)	If the above agent is ineffective, concomitantly use one of the following agents • LABA[a] (a compounding agent can be used) • LTRA • Theophylline sustained-release preparation	Concomitantly use one or more of the agents below • LABA[a] (a compounding agent can be used) • LTRA • Theophylline sustained-release preparation • LAMA	Concomitantly use multiple agents of those • LABA[a] (a compounding agent can be used) • LTRA • Theophylline sustained-release preparation • LAMA • Anti-IgE antibody • OCS
	Additional treatment	Anti-allergics other than LTRA	Anti-allergics other than LTRA	Anti-allergics other than LTRA	Anti-allergics other than LTRA
Exacerbation treatment[b]		Inhaled SABA	Inhaled SABA	Inhaled SABA	Inhaled SABA

GINA for long-term management					
	Step 1	**Step 2**	**Step 3**	**Step 4**	**Step 5**
Preferred controller choice	None	Low dose ICS	Low dose ICS/LABA	Med/high ICS/LABA	Refer for add-on treatment (e.g., LAMA[c], anti-IgE, anti-IL-5)
Other controller options	Consider low dose ICS	LTRA Low dose theophylline	Med/high dose ICS Low dose ICS+LTRA (or +theophylline)	Add tiotropium[c] High dose ICS + LTRA (or +theophylline)	Add low dose OCS
Reliever	As-needed SABA		As-needed SABA or low dose ICS/formeterol[d]		

LTRA leukotriene receptor antagonists, *LABA* long-acting β2 agonist, *SABA* short-acting β2 agonist, *LAMA* long-acting muscarinic antagonist, *OCS* oral corticosteroids

[a]In patients treated with a combination of budesonide/formoterol as a controller, if used as a rescue agent, it should not be used beyond the maximum number of uses per time and per day. The maximum number of uses is generally up to 8 inhalations/day; however, temporarily, it can be used for up to 12 inhalations/day (for 3 days: budesonide, 1920 mg/day; formoterol 54 mg/day). When more than 8 inhalations/day of budesonide/formoterol are needed, a physician should be consulted

[b]Management against mild exacerbations is shown. For other exacerbations, refer to Table 11.5

[c]Tiotropium by mist inhaler is an add-on treatment for patients with a history of exacerbations

[d]Low dose ICS/formoterol is the reliever medication for patients prescribed low dose budesonide/formoterol or low dose beclomethasone/formoterol maintenance and reliever therapy

Table 11.3 Selection of treatment steps based on symptoms of untreated patients in JGL 2017 [1]

Selection of treatment step		Treatment step 1	Treatment step 2	Treatment step 3	Treatment step 4
Correspondent severity[a]		Mild intermittent	Mild persistent	Moderate persistent	Severe persistent
Features of asthma symptoms	Frequency	Less than once a week	Once or more a week, not every day	Every day	Every day
	Intensity	Mild and brief	Disturbs daily life or sleep at least once a month	Disturbs daily life or sleep at least once a week	Restricts daily life
				Need for SABA use almost every day	Worsens frequently even under treatment
	Symptoms at night	Less than twice a month	Twice or more a month	Once or more a week	Frequently

[a]Determine the severity based on the presence of any one of the features

combined with an ICS has been reported [7]. Bronchial thermoplasty (BT) is an emerging intervention for severe asthma that delivers thermal energy to the airway wall through a dedicated catheter to reduce the airway smooth muscle (ASM) mass [8]. BT has been approved since 2015 in Japan and is listed in both guidelines as an alternative treatment option.

11.3.3 Stepwise Approach for Initial Treatment

For the initial treatment of untreated asthmatics, the intensity of asthma treatment (treatment step) is determined based on the asthma symptoms (Table 11.3). Especially, symptom-based severity is often applicable in clinical practice as follows. (1) Mild intermittent: symptoms that do not occur every week; (2) mild persistent: symptoms that occur every week, but not every day; (3) moderate persistent: symptoms that occur every day, but do not disturb daily life; (4) severe persistent: symptoms that occur every day and disturb daily life (Table 11.3). Once the severity is determined, treatment steps are determined as follows: step 1 treatment for mild intermittent symptoms, step 2 treatment for mild persistent symptoms, step 3 treatment for moderate persistent symptoms; and step 4 treatment for severe persistent symptoms. In asthmatics under treatment, the treatment steps are determined by both the asthmatic symptoms and the content of the current asthma treatment (Table 11.4).

In essence, low dose ICS is the main controller at every step in JGL. When asthma attacks occur during management, a SABA should be used as a reliever. In steps 2 and 3, if patients are treated with a combination of budesonide and for-

Table 11.4 Classification of asthma severity based on the present treatment (adults) in JGL 2017[1]

Patient's symptoms in the present treatment	Treatment step 1	Treatment step 2	Treatment step 3	Treatment step 4
Controlled[a] • No symptoms • No symptoms at night	Mild intermittent	Mild persistent	Moderate persistent	Severe persistent
Mild intermittent[b] • Less than once a week • Mild and brief • Less than twice a month at night	Mild intermittent	Mild persistent	Moderate persistent	Severe persistent
Mild persistent[c] • Once or more a week, not every day • Once or more a month, disturbs everyday life and sleep • Twice or more a month at night	Mild persistent	Moderate persistent	Severe persistent	Severe persistent
Moderate persistent[c] • Every day • Requires short-acting inhaled b2 agonist almost every day • Once or more a week, disturbs everyday life and sleep • Once or more a week at night	Moderate persistent	Severe persistent	Severe persistent	Most severe persistent
Severe persistent[c] • Frequently exacerbated even under treatment • Every day • Restricts everyday life • Frequently occurs at night	Severe persistent	Severe persistent	Severe persistent	Most severe persistent

[a]Consider step-down after continued treatment for 3–6 months
[b]Enhance treatment at each step
[c]Check adherence to treatment, and consider step-up as needed

moterol as a controller, its use as a reliever can be approved (SMART: Single maintenance and reliever therapy). The details of each step are as follows (Table 11.2).

11.3.3.1 Step 1 Treatment: One or No Controller Agent Plus Reliever Agent

A low dose of an ICS is recommended to use as a basic controller. Use of a SABA without ICS should be limited to patients with rare occurrence of asthma symptoms (less than once a month). For patients whose symptoms occur once or more a month, a low dose ICS is recommended as a controller agent because low grade inflammation exists even in the airways of mild asthmatics [9]. If ICSs cannot be used, LTRAs [10] or sustained-release theophylline [11] can be an alternative controller.

Anti-allergics other than LTRAs such as a histamine H1 blocker, thromboxane A2 inhibitors, and Th2 cytokine inhibitors can be used, according to the pathophysiology of the asthma.

11.3.3.2 Step 2 Treatment: Two Controller Agents Plus a Reliever Agent

In addition to ICSs (low to medium dose), use of LABA is recommended [12, 13]. ICSs plus LABAs are considered to be more effective than moderate doses of ICS monotherapy [14]. Furthermore, the ICS/LABA combination preparation has a superior effect compared to ICS plus LABA prescribed in separate inhalers [15]. LTRA [16, 17] or sustained-release theophylline [18] can be used with patients who cannot use LABAs. Early treatment with ICS/LABA can rapidly improve asthmatic symptoms and pulmonary function compared to ICS monotherapy [14, 15]. LTRAs are useful mainly in patients with coexisting allergic rhinitis and exercise- or aspirin-induced asthma.

11.3.3.3 Step 3 Treatment: Two or More Controller Agents Plus a Reliever Agent

The combination of ICS (medium to high dose) with a LABA is recommended. If the effects of an ICS/LABA are insufficient, either an LTRA, a sustained-release theophylline, or LAMA is concomitantly used with ICS/LABA.

11.3.3.4 Step 4 Treatment: Controller Agents Plus Additional Therapy Plus Reliever Agent

In addition to continuous use of high dose of ICS and LABA, an LTRA, sustained-release theophylline, and/or LAMA are used. In poorly controlled patients using all of the controllers, anti-IgE antibody (omalizumab) is shown to be effective if the patients are sensitized to perennial allergens, and whose serum total IgE is within a therapeutic target range (30–1500 IU/mL) [19]. The dose of the anti-IgE antibody is dependent on a dosage conversion table. The effectiveness is evaluated 16 weeks after administration and, if effective, patients receive continuous administration. If it is not effective, this pharmacotherapy should be withdrawn. Oral corticosteroids (OCS) should be intermittently administered for a short period to avoid prolonged use. Specifically, around 0.5 mg/kg or the equivalent amount of prednisolone is administered for a short period (usually less than 1 week), and a high-dose ICS is subsequently used. In patients with insufficient asthma control, who need continuous administration of OCS, a shorter-acting OCS (prednisolone) can be administered every day or every other day in the morning to maintain the minimum dose (5 mg). In the step 4 patients with eosinophilia in the peripheral blood, anti-IL-5 antibody (mepolizumab) can be used.

In contrast to the JGL, a stepwise approach is not used for the initial treatment in GINA. The initial controller for untreated patients is determined based on the presenting symptoms and frequency of SABA use in GINA. Notably, a controller is not recommended for patients without asthma symptoms or with a need for SABA less than twice a month in GINA. In contrast, low dose ICS use is basically recommended in all steps in the Japanese guidelines because low grade inflammation exists even in the airways of mild asthmatics.

11.3.4 Stepwise Approach for Long-Term Management

In patients who have already taken pharmacotherapy, such as controllers for asthma treatment, the severity is determined based on the remaining symptoms under the current step (Table 11.4). When symptoms are still uncontrolled in patients treated with step 3 treatment, they should consult a specialist. In general, the control status should be assessed within 1 month of the initial treatment regarding the symptoms, frequency of reliever use, limitations in daily life, pulmonary function, and asthma exacerbations. In addition, the inhaler technique, adherence, side-effects, understanding of the treatment plan, and patient satisfaction need to be reviewed. When symptoms still exist less than once a week, intensification of the treatment within the same treatment step should be considered. When asthma symptoms occur every week or every day, 1 step-up or 2 steps-up are required. A step-down should be considered if the asthma control status remains good for 3–6 months. It is important to repeat assessment of the control status and adjustment of the treatment every 1–3 months because the goal of asthma treatment is to maintain good asthma control using a minimum of drugs.

For long-term management, a stepwise approach is used also in GINA. The treatment steps for long-term management are divided into five steps and no controller is recommended in the step 1 treatment as for the initial treatment (Table 11.2) This suggests that the JGL highlight the importance of improving chronic airway inflammation for long-term management of asthma because the final goal of treatment in the Japanese guideline is "no symptoms."

11.4 Management of Acute Exacerbation

11.4.1 Management at Home

As the severity of asthma symptoms varies widely among patients, each patient requires a clear indication of the approach for managing asthma exacerbations based on the individual severity. For this purpose, an action plan with specific instructions for each condition (a written document for self-management) should be provided to each patient [20]. For example, when patients have wheezing/chest tightness and moderate asthma symptoms, 1–2 puffs of a SABA in pressurized metered-dose inhaler (pMDI) should be administered. If insufficient, inhalation can be repeated every 20 min for 1 h, and then once an hour. Patients under single inhaler maintenance and reliever therapy (SMART) using BUD/FM can inhale BUD/FM once for exacerbations. If the exacerbation does not improve within a few minutes, 1 more inhalation can be added [21]. Patients can continue treatment at home when the symptoms disappear with these approaches and their effects persist for 3–4 h. However, if their effects are insufficient, patients should take oral prednisolone at 15–30 mg, and immediate referral to an emergency outpatient is necessary.

11.4.2 Treatment Procedures in Emergency Outpatients

On arrival at the emergency outpatient clinic, the severity should be immediately determined by symptoms as follows: (1) mild: dyspnea without difficulty in lying down; (2) moderate: difficulty in lying down and walking; (3) severe: abasia, difficulty in moving and speaking; and (4) serious symptoms: cyanosis, impaired consciousness, and respiratory arrest. PEF, SpO_2, PaO_2, and $PaCO_2$ should be measured immediately to assess the exacerbation intensity. However, the main determinant of severity is the degree of dyspnea. Treatment steps for exacerbations are classified into four steps (Table 11.5) and selected based on the severity.

The following are general outlines of treatment for each grade of severity (also summarized in Table 11.5).

11.4.2.1 Wheezing/Chest Tightness, Mild Symptoms (Mild Exacerbations)

At first, the step 1 treatment should be started by inhalation of SABA. If symptoms disappear and are stable for 60 min without additional treatment, confirm that there is no airway obstruction (%PEF ≥80%) and discharge the patient. If improvement of symptoms is insufficient and airway obstruction persists (%PEF <80%), the patients should be treated by the step 2 treatment.

11.4.2.2 Moderate Symptoms and Continuous Mild Symptoms (Moderate Exacerbation)

The patients should be treated by the step 2 treatment.

1. Patients should inhale SABA using a nebulizer repeatedly every 20–30 min until symptoms improve. If symptoms improve within 60 min and are stable for 60 min after the last inhalation with 95% or higher of SpO_2, the patient can be discharged. If improvement is insufficient, the following treatments should be started.

Table 11.5 Treatment steps for asthma exacerbation [1]

	Treatment	Home remedy, emergency visit and hospitalization, and ICU treatment
Treatment step 1	Inhaled short-acting β2-agonist (SABA) Additional inhalation of budesonide/formoterol, as needed[a]	Home remedy
Treatment step 2	Repeated inhalation of SABA using a nebulizer[b] Intravenous drip infusion of aminophylline[c] Oxygen (target SpO2 at 95%) Systemic administration of steroid[d] Inhaled anticholinergics Subcutaneous injection of Bosmin®(adrenaline, 0.1%)[e]	Emergency visit – If symptoms improve within 1 h, the patient may be discharged – Insufficient responses within 2–4 h – No response within 1–2 h Hospital admission: switch to treatment step 3 as for severe exacerbation
Treatment step 3	Repeated inhalation of SABA using a nebulizer[b] Repeated administration of systemic steroid[d] Oxygen (target SpO_2 at 95%) Intravenous drip infusion of aminophylline (continuous)[f] Inhaled anticholinergics Subcutaneous injection of Bosmin®(adrenaline, 0.1%)[e]	Emergency visit If no response within 1 h, hospitalization If exacerbated, switch to treatment for serious exacerbation
Treatment step 4	Continue the above treatment If symptoms and respiratory function are exacerbated, conduct intubation[g] Despite oxygen inhalation, ≤50 mmHg PaO_2 and/or rapidly elevated $PaCO_2$ with impaired consciousness Mechanical ventilation,[g] Bronchial lavage Consider general anesthesia (using isoflurane, sevoflurane, etc.)	Immediate hospitalization and ICU treatment[g]

Aim of treatment: elimination of dyspnea, normal movement, normal sleep, and normal everyday life. PEF rate is ≥80% of the predicted value or the best value. Oxygen saturation >95% (values after bronchodilator administration). No exacerbation of asthma symptoms by routine medication and inhalation

Consider treatment step-up when the aim of treatment cannot be achieved within 1 h

[a]Repeat 1–2 puffs of SABA pMDI twice at an interval of 20 min

[b]Inhalation of SABA using a nebulizer: repeat every 20–30 min. Monitor the pulse, which should be maintained at ≤130/min

[c]Intravenous drip infusion of aminophylline (6 mg/kg) in 200–250 mL of isotonic fluid: Administer for about 1 h. If adverse reactions occur, discontinue the infusion. When a sufficient amount of theophylline had been administered before exacerbation, reduce the dose of aminophylline to half or less. Routinely, measure serum theophylline levels in patients receiving this drug whenever possible

[d]Intravenous drip infusion of steroids: intravenous drip infusion of 200–500 mg of hydrocortisone, 40–125 mg of methylprednisolone, or 4–8 mg of dexamethasone or betamethasone. Subsequently,

(continued)

Table 11.5 (continued)

conduct intravenous drip infusion of 100–200 mg of hydrocortisone, or 40–80 mg of methylprednisolone every 4–6 h as needed, or 4–8 mg of dexamethasone or betamethasone every 6 h as needed, or oral prednisolone (0.5 mg/kg/day). Steroid succinate esters (i.e., methyl prednisolone, prednisolone sodium succinate) should be avoided in patients who have or are suspected of having aspirin-induced asthma

[e]Bosmin® (adrenaline, 0.1%): Bosmin® (0.1–0.3 mL) can be repeatedly administered at intervals of 20–30 min. Monitor the pulse to be maintained at ≤130/min. This agent is contraindicated in patients with ischemic heart disease, glaucoma (except for open-angle [simple] glaucoma), and hyperthyroidism. Sphygmomanometry and electrocardiography are required for patients with hypertension

[f]Continuous intravenous infusion of aminophylline: following the first intravenous infusion (see footnote "e"), conduct continuous intravenous infusion of 250 mg of aminophylline for 5–7 h (about 0.6–0.8 mg/kg/h). Monitor serum theophylline levels which should be maintained at 10–20 mg/mL (15–20 mg/mL to achieve the maximum effects). If adverse reactions occur, discontinue the infusion

[g]ICU or hospital rooms where tracheal intubation, assisted ventilation, bronchial lavage, etc. can be performed and continuous monitoring can be conducted using a sphygmomanometer, electrocardiogram, and pulse oximeter. Since intubation and mechanical ventilation during severe respiratory insufficiency are often life-threatening, they should be used by experienced specialists when inevitable in emergency

2. Systemic steroid (200–500 mg of hydrocortisone, 40–125 mg of methylprednisolone, or 4–8 mg of dexamethasone or betamethasone) should be administered immediately through intravenous drip infusion in cases of moderate or more severe exacerbations or poor response to the initial SABA inhalation. Patients taking a high dose ICS (equivalent to fluticasone propionate (FP) ≥800 μg/day) or an oral corticosteroid as a controller, or are in a high-risk asthmatic group should also receive intravenous administration of systemic steroid [22]. Steroid succinate esters (hydrocortisone or methylprednisolone) should be avoided for patients with or suspected of aspirin-exacerbated respiratory disease (AERD). Slow, intravenous infusion for about an hour is recommended for patients with unconfirmed AERD, or patients who are receiving the agent for the first time.
3. Nasal administration of oxygenation at a dose of 1–2 L should be started for patients with SpO_2 less than 95% (PaO_2 <80 mmHg), or with symptoms suggesting hypoxemia.
4. Six mg/kg of aminophylline in 200–250 mL of isotonic fluid is administered through intravenous drip infusion.
5. Anticholinergics can be added if the treatment effect described above is insufficient.
6. If the symptoms remain, a physician needs to consider subcutaneous injection of 0.1–0.3 mL of adrenaline (0.1%). Adrenaline can be injected repeatedly at intervals of 20–30 min (not to exceed 130 beats per min in pulse rate).

When symptoms improve (i.e., wheezing and dyspnea are absent for 1 h), such patients can be discharged. At discharge, the patients need a step-up of the long-term treatment. When the response is insufficient (mild wheezing and dyspnea remain) or no response is observed, step 3 treatment should be considered. When symptoms do not improve within 1–2 h, hospitalization should be considered. After hospitalization, continue step 3 treatment.

11.4.2.3 Severe Symptoms (Severe Exacerbations) or Continued Moderate Symptoms

The patients should be treated by the step 2 treatment followed by step 3 for continuous treatment.

(1) Initial treatment: obtain venous access promptly and start step 2 treatment as outlined below.

a. Administration of SABA using a nebulizer.
b. Intravenous drip infusion of corticosteroids.
c. Oxygen administration. Targeted PaO_2 is approximately 80 mmHg (SpO_2 95%) with attention to prevent CO_2 narcosis. Noninvasive positive-pressure ventilation (NPPV), endotracheal intubation, and mechanical ventilation should be considered in patients with a poor response.
d. Intravenous drip infusion of aminophylline.
e. Subcutaneous injection of adrenaline.

If symptoms do not improve within 1 h, consider hospitalization.

(2) Continuous treatment

The patients are initially treated by step 2 treatment and need to continue step 3 treatment.

a. Repeated administration of systemic corticosteroids.

An oral prednisolone (approximately 0.5 mg/kg/day) once in the morning can also be administered and can be discontinued or reduced to the usual dose by 7–14 days after remission. Tapering the dose of an oral corticosteroid has no benefit [23]. Patients can start ICS when their breathing difficulties improve.

b. Oxygen.

The targeted oxygenation (SpO_2 95%, PaO_2 80 mmHg) needs to be maintained.

c. Continuous intravenous drip infusion of aminophylline.

Continuous intravenous drip infusion of aminophylline at a dose of 0.6–0.8 mg/kg/h is recommended to reduce symptoms. The serum level of aminophylline should be kept at 8–20 μg/mL. If adverse reactions develop, discontinue the administration immediately and measure the serum theophylline levels.

11.4.2.4 Serious Asthma Symptoms and Emergency (Serious Exacerbations)

The patients should be treated with step 4 treatment as outlined below.

1. Endotracheal intubation and mechanical ventilation [24]
2. Treatment for exacerbation: 0.3–1.0 mL of SABA or adrenaline (0.1% before dilution), both diluted 10 times with physiological saline, can be administered

through an endotracheal tube. Patients should be initially and continuously treated by step 3 treatment. Consider general anesthesia using a narcotic agent (isoflurane, sevoflurane, and others) for refractory symptoms, because these agents have bronchodilatory activity. The use of halothane should be avoided.

Similar to the home management plan for acute exacerbations in the JGL, GINA recommends providing self-management education of worsening asthma for all asthmatic patients. In contrast to the JGL, the management of acute exacerbations at an outpatient department is different in the primary care and emergency departments. In any setting, inhaled SABA is a key medication for the treatment of an acute exacerbation of asthma. In the JGL, stepwise treatment is recommended, in contrast to GINA. There are some differences in the treatment options between both guidelines. In the GINA guidelines, intramuscular epinephrine is indicated only for acute asthma related to anaphylaxis and angioedema and it is not routinely used for other asthma exacerbations. In addition, GINA does not recommend intravenous aminophylline in view of its poor efficacy and safety profile.

11.5 Conclusions

This chapter provides an overview of the treatment of asthma for long-term management and acute exacerbations in the JGL. The remarkable characteristics of the Japanese guidelines are that (1) low dose of ICS is recommended in step 1 treatment for initial treatment and long-term management of asthma, (2) the goal of treatment is "no symptoms," and (3) treatment steps are explicit for both long-term management and acute exacerbations. There are some differences between the two guidelines as mentioned above. Hopefully, understanding of the JGL will be helpful for many physicians to treat and manage all asthmatic patients.

References

1. Ichinose M, Sugiura H, Nagase H, Yamaguchi M, Inoue H, Sagara H, et al. Japanese guidelines for adult asthma 2017. Allergol Int. 2017;66(2):163–89.
2. Global Initiative for Asthma. Global Strategy for Asthma Management and Prevention; 2017. Available from: www.ginasthma.org.
3. Ohashi Y, Motojima S, Fukuda T, Makino S. Airway hyperresponsiveness, increased intracellular spaces of bronchial epithelium, and increased infiltration of eosinophils and lymphocytes in bronchial mucosa in asthma. Am Rev Respir Dis. 1992;145(6):1469–76.
4. Bousquet J, Chanez P, Lacoste JY, Barneon G, Ghavanian N, Enander I, et al. Eosinophilic inflammation in asthma. N Engl J Med. 1990;323(15):1033–9.

5. Vignola AM, Chanez P, Campbell AM, Souques F, Lebel B, Enander I, et al. Airway inflammation in mild intermittent and in persistent asthma. Am J Respir Crit Care Med. 1998;157(2):403–9.
6. Roche WR, Beasley R, Williams JH, Holgate ST. Subepithelial fibrosis in the bronchi of asthmatics. Lancet. 1989;1(8637):520–4.
7. Tamura G, Sano Y, Hirata K, Ishioka S, Nakashima M, Miyamoto T. Effect of transdermal tulobuterol added to inhaled corticosteroids in asthma patients. Allergol Int. 2005;54(4): 615–20.
8. Castro M, Rubin AS, Laviolette M, Fiterman J, De Andrade Lima M, Shah PL, et al. Effectiveness and safety of bronchial thermoplasty in the treatment of severe asthma: a multicenter, randomized, double-blind, sham-controlled clinical trial. Am J Respir Crit Care Med. 2010;181(2):116–24.
9. Pauwels RA, Pedersen S, Busse WW, Tan WC, Chen YZ, Ohlsson SV, et al. Early intervention with budesonide in mild persistent asthma: a randomised, double-blind trial. Lancet. 2003;361(9363):1071–6.
10. Drazen JM, Israel E, O'Byrne PM. Treatment of asthma with drugs modifying the leukotriene pathway. N Engl J Med. 1999;340(3):197–206.
11. Sullivan P, Bekir S, Jaffar Z, Page C, Jeffery P, Costello J. Anti-inflammatory effects of low-dose oral theophylline in atopic asthma. Lancet. 1994;343(8904):1006–8.
12. Lemanske RF Jr, Sorkness CA, Mauger EA, Lazarus SC, Boushey HA, Fahy JV, et al. Inhaled corticosteroid reduction and elimination in patients with persistent asthma receiving salmeterol: a randomized controlled trial. JAMA. 2001;285(20):2594–603.
13. Greening AP, Ind PW, Northfield M, Shaw G, Allen & Hanburys Limited UK Study Group. Added salmeterol versus higher-dose corticosteroid in asthma patients with symptoms on existing inhaled corticosteroid. Lancet. 1994;344(8917):219–24.
14. Matsunaga K, Kawabata H, Hirano T, Sugiura H, Minakata Y, Ichinose M. Difference in time-course of improvement in asthma control measures between budesonide and budesonide/formoterol. Pulm Pharmacol Ther. 2013;26(2):189–94.
15. Bateman ED, Boushey HA, Bousquet J, Busse WW, Clark TJ, Pauwels RA, et al. Can guideline-defined asthma control be achieved? The gaining optimal asthma control study. Am J Respir Crit Care Med. 2004;170(8):836–44.
16. Bjermer L, Bisgaard H, Bousquet J, Fabbri LM, Greening AP, Haahtela T, et al. Montelukast and fluticasone compared with salmeterol and fluticasone in protecting against asthma exacerbation in adults: one year, double blind, randomised, comparative trial. BMJ. 2003;3 27(7420):891.
17. Nelson HS, Busse WW, Kerwin E, Church N, Emmett A, Rickard K, et al. Fluticasone propionate/salmeterol combination provides more effective asthma control than low-dose inhaled corticosteroid plus montelukast. J Allergy Clin Immunol. 2000;106(6): 1088–95.
18. Evans DJ, Taylor DA, Zetterstrom O, Chung KF, O'Connor BJ, Barnes PJ. A comparison of low-dose inhaled budesonide plus theophylline and high-dose inhaled budesonide for moderate asthma. N Engl J Med. 1997;337(20):1412–8.
19. Humbert M, Beasley R, Ayres J, Slavin R, Hebert J, Bousquet J, et al. Benefits of omalizumab as add-on therapy in patients with severe persistent asthma who are inadequately controlled despite best available therapy (GINA 2002 step 4 treatment): INNOVATE. Allergy. 2005;60(3):309–16.
20. Beasley R, Cushley M, Holgate ST. A self management plan in the treatment of adult asthma. Thorax. 1989;44(3):200–4.
21. Bousquet J, Boulet LP, Peters MJ, Magnussen H, Quiralte J, Martinez-Aguilar NE, et al. Budesonide/formoterol for maintenance and relief in uncontrolled asthma vs. high-dose salmeterol/fluticasone. Respir Med. 2007;101(12):2437–46.

22. Turner MO, Noertjojo K, Vedal S, Bai T, Crump S, Fitzgerald JM. Risk factors for near-fatal asthma. A case-control study in hospitalized patients with asthma. Am J Respir Crit Care Med. 1998;157(6 Pt 1):1804–9.
23. O'Driscoll BR, Kalra S, Wilson M, Pickering CA, Carroll KB, Woodcock AA. Double-blind trial of steroid tapering in acute asthma. Lancet. 1993;341(8841):324–7.
24. Darioli R, Perret C. Mechanical controlled hypoventilation in status asthmaticus. Am Rev Respir Dis. 1984;129(3):385–7.

Chapter 12
How to Improve Adherence Technique for Inhaler Use and Selection of Inhalers

Takahiko Horiguchi and Rieko Kondo

Abstract Unlike oral medication, inhalants have the drawback that there is no therapeutic effect if the drug does not reach the bronchi. It is essential that doctors select appropriate inhalants suited to the patient and that instruction on correct inhalation technique is provided. This article provides an overview of the characteristics and selection method of the 12 different devices currently available in Japan, as well as the specific methods and technique for proper inhalation instruction.

Keyword Inhalation instruction · Inhaled steroids · Inhalant selection method · Inhalation instruction DVD · Tongue position during inhalation

12.1 Introduction

Inhalant medication is the first-line therapy for bronchial asthma [1, 2]. Currently in Japan, 12 types of inhalant devices are covered by insurance; the different characteristics of the drugs and devices are complicated, and there are no clear selection criteria for patients with different backgrounds, making selection difficult for non-specialist doctors. The complexity of the inhalation instructions is also problematic [3–7], and the need for new tools has been indicated [8]. Unlike oral medication, if inhalants are not correctly delivered from the device to the bronchial area, the desired effect will not be achieved, which leads to the risk of unnecessary step-up. It is important not only to have device operations that can be checked visually, as is the norm, but also those that can be monitored in areas where a visual check is impossible, including the state of the drug in the mouth and the position of the

T. Horiguchi (✉) · R. Kondo
Department of Respiratory Medicine II, Fujita Health University School of Medicine, Nagoya, Aichi, Japan
e-mail: ta-hori@fujita-hu.ac.jp

A. Yokoyama (ed.), *Advances in Asthma*, Respiratory Disease Series: Diagnostic Tools and Disease Managements, https://doi.org/10.1007/978-981-13-2790-2_12

tongue. To ensure that all medical facilities throughout Japan receive standardized inhalation instructions, we have created a poster and a DVD, containing audio and video recordings of the operating procedures and main instruction points for the 12 different devices available in Japan [9]. Here we summarize instruction methods that allow patients to master the techniques efficiently within a limited timeframe.

12.2 Device Types and Characteristics

12.2.1 Pressurized Metered-Dose Inhaler (pMDI)

Within the pMDI category, there is the solution type (type of inhaler where the particles are already dissolved in liquid, and it is not necessary to shake the aluminum can before use) and the suspension type (type of inhaler where fine particles are dispersed within the liquid, making it necessary to shake the aluminum can before use), but these represent a single type of device, with essentially the same operating method. While inhalation of the sprayed aerosol is not affected by inspiratory force, it is necessary to synchronize breath intake with the spray. Patients who find it difficult to synchronize their breath intake (elderly patients, patients with dementia, patients with disuse changes, patients unable to maintain a seated position, patients with neuromuscular disorders, etc.) are able to use these devices by using a spacer or with assistance. With a spacer, the large particles adhere to the auxiliary tool, which reduces the level of adhesion to the inside of the mouth, and thus should also reduce the adverse drug reactions. pMDI preparations float in the air with Brownian motion, which lengthens the duration of time in the air, making it easier for the drug to reach the peripheral airways. The solution type of inhaled corticosteroid (ICS), in particular (Qvar®, Alvesco®), has a small average particle size of approximately 1 μm, making it suitable for patients with residual lesions in the peripheral airways. Depending on the product, some have an alcohol odor, while for others it is difficult to check the remaining quantity; therefore, caution is needed.

12.2.2 Dry Powder Inhaler (DPI)

There are nine different types of DPI devices, and each has different operating procedures; care is therefore needed to prevent the inhalation instructions becoming overcomplicated. With DPI, the drug is absorbed with spontaneous breathing, so that synchronized breathing is not required, but it does require a certain level of inspiratory flow rate. DPI does not require a propellant; thus, there is no odor of alcohol. However, because a powder is inhaled, it can irritate the throat, and some patients can choke with this medication. This is seen particularly often in young women; therefore, these patients should consider switching to a preparation with a smaller particle diameter or to a pMDI preparation.

1. Diskhaler: Flutide® (ICS), Serevent® (long-acting β2 agonist, LABA)

   Released in Japan in 1998 as the first DPI device. It was divided into four blister packs, and exchanging these was time-consuming; it was therefore replaced with a disk from 2002. The anti-influenza drug Relenza® has the same device configuration.

2. Discus: Flutide® (ICS), Adoair® (ICS/LABA compound), Serevent® (LABA)
   Easy to operate, resulting in few operating errors. The mean particle diameter is approximately 3.2 μm, which is comparatively large, and the amount inhaled per dose is 12.5 mg, which is also relatively large.
3. Turbuhaler: Pulmicort® (ICS), Symbicort® (ICS/LABA compound)
   The mean particle diameter is small, at approximately 2.2–2.7 μm, and the amount inhaled per dose is also small, at 0.89 mg, which helps to prevent choking. Symbicort® has treatment steps 2 and 3, and if up to eight inhalation doses per day are used, it is possible to use SMART (Symbicort maintenance and reliever therapy) during an attack.
4. Twisthaler: Asmanex® (ICS)
   The mean particle diameter is approximately 2.5 μm, which is small for a DPI, and it easily reaches the peripheral airways. The device is filled by simply opening the cap, making it easy to use. When the device is empty, it locks and cannot be reopened, making it clear when the medication has been depleted.
5. Ellipta: Relvar® (ICS)
   The device enables inhalation with a single action, making it extremely easy to use. It requires one dose per day, making it superior in terms of adherence. However, the mean particle diameter is large, at 4.0 μm (fluticasone), and the inhaled amount per dose is also large, at 25 mg; hence, it must be used with caution in patients prone to choking.
6. Swinghaler: Meptin® (short-acting β2 agonist, SABA)
   The only DPI preparation among the short-acting β2 agonists.

12.2.3 Soft Mist Inhaler (SMI)

1. SMI: Spiriva® Respimat® (long-acting muscarinic antagonist, LAMA)
   SMIs have a slow ejection, over approximately 1.5 s, so that it can be inhaled by patients who cannot achieve adequate inspiratory flow rate and by patients who find it difficult to synchronize their breath, making it a superior device. However, the preparation is complicated and requires some strength, and therefore, having the device set by a pharmacist would be ideal.

12.2.4 Suspension: Pulmicort® (ICS)

1. Inhaled using a nebulizer. Suitable for patients who find it difficult to inhale even using a spacer with a mask (infants, children, elderly, etc.). A jet-type (compressor) nebulizer is suitable for this device, but it is not covered by insurance.

In patients prescribed multiple devices, it should be noted that the patients may confuse the usage methods and number of inhalations; thus, caution is needed. The problems and countermeasures for each device have been compiled in Fig. 12.1 [10].

		Problems	Solutions
pMDI	BDP, CIC	Difficult to synchronize	Use a spacer
	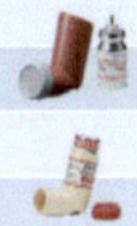	Too weak to push	Use auxiliary equipment
		Difficult to determine the remaining amount	Use a residual amount meter
		Alcohol sensitivity	Switch to alcohol-free preparation
		Hold upside down to inhale	Inhalation instruction
DPI	FP, SF	Mouthpiece is flat, difficult to fit lips around it	Select a device that fits the mouth easily
	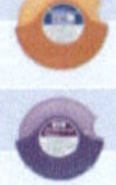	Insufficient inspiratory flowrate	Check and practice with the discus trainer*1
		Choking due to large particle size	Select medication with smaller particle diameter
		Relatively high rate of local adverse reactions	Thoroughly instruct and check the gargling method
		Unable to see the counter numbers, hence continue to use even when it has reached zero	Provide instructions for checking the residual amount counter by using a dedicated magnifying lens
	BUD, FBC	Tilt or hold horizontally when twisting	Instruct to hold vertical
	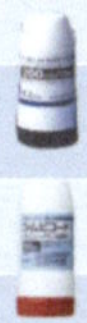	Do not understand or forget the empty space when twisting	Make an agreement with the pharmacist to do this task
		Cannot understand the twisting	Explain that twisting can be either from the right or the left direction, but the device needs to be twisted until it stops
		It makes a noise when shaken, which is mistaken as residual medication	Explain the sound of the desiccant
		It is difficult to understand how to determine the remaining medication	Affix a remaining medication check sticker to BUD
		Cannot maintain inspiratory flowrate	Check and practice with a Turbutester*2
		Does not feel like the medication has been inhaled	Communicate information during inhalation instruction
		The clip is small and tends to be slippery	Fit a grip supporter*3
	MF	Tilt or hold horizontally when twisting (easy to tilt while looking at the counter)	Instruct to hold vertical
	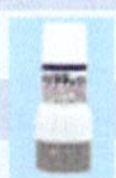	Cannot maintain inspiratory flowrate	Check with In-Check*4
		Round mouthpiece makes it difficult to inhale	Select a device that fits the mouth better
		The cap does not open smoothly	Inhalation instruction
		Inadequate cap closure means the next dose does not fill	Instruct to close firmly until the click is heard

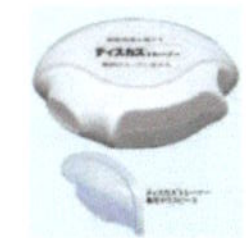

*1 Discus trainer

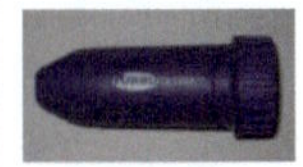

*2 Turbu tester

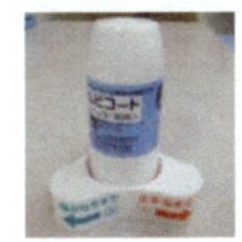

*3 Grip supporter

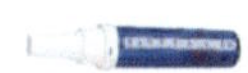

*4 In-Check

Fig. 12.1 Inhalant problems and solutions

Disk type		Problems	Solutions
DPI	Ellipta 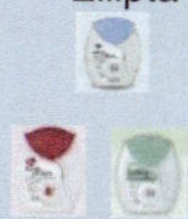	Tendency to choke with the large particle size and a single large dose	This complaint is particularly common in young women. Switch to medication with a finer particle size
		Hard to open the lid	Open until there is a click sound
		Insufficient inspiratory flowrate	Check and practice with discus trainer
		Relatively high rate of local adverse reactions	Thoroughly instruct and check the gargling method
	Breezhaler 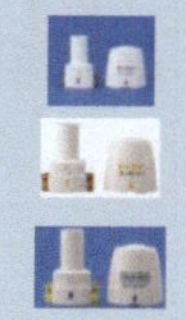	Aluminium sheet is difficult to remove (Seebri®, Ultibro®)	Ask the pharmacist to peel a part of the sheet in order to make it easier to remove
		Inhale without opening the hole	Check the inhalation technique
		Press the button numerous times	Take care because the capsule will be damaged
		Powder causes choking	Investigate changing devices
		Does not make a clattering sound during inhalation	Lightly shake the container and inhale again
		Medication remaining in the capsule	Instruct to inhale repeatedly until the medicine has completely been inhaled
	Eklira 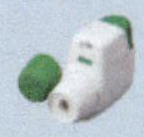	Inhale twice a day	Check continued compliance
		The mouthpiece is round, large, and smooth, hence cannot bite lightly with teeth	Instruct to hold it as deeply as possible in the mouth and lower the tongue
		Mouthpiece is round and large, so the tongue tends to sit directly in front	Instruct to hold as deeply as possible in the mouth and lower the tongue
SMI	Respimat 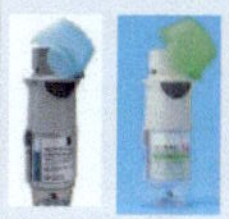	Priming is complicated	Request the pharmacist to prime the device
		Cartridge is hard to load	Request the pharmacist to prime the device
		Hard to turn 180 degrees	Use an auxiliary device (*Kaiten-kun* [Rotation-helper])
		Fills without closing the cap	Easy to mis-spray
		Spray without holding firmly in mouth (mistakenly use open-mouth method)	Take care to ensure the medication does not enter the eyes, as it is anticholinergic medication
		Priming is complicated after not using for sometime	Use after performing a test spray. After 7 days of non-use (1 spray), and after 21 days of non-use (3 sprays after seeing the mist)

Fig. 12.1 (continued)

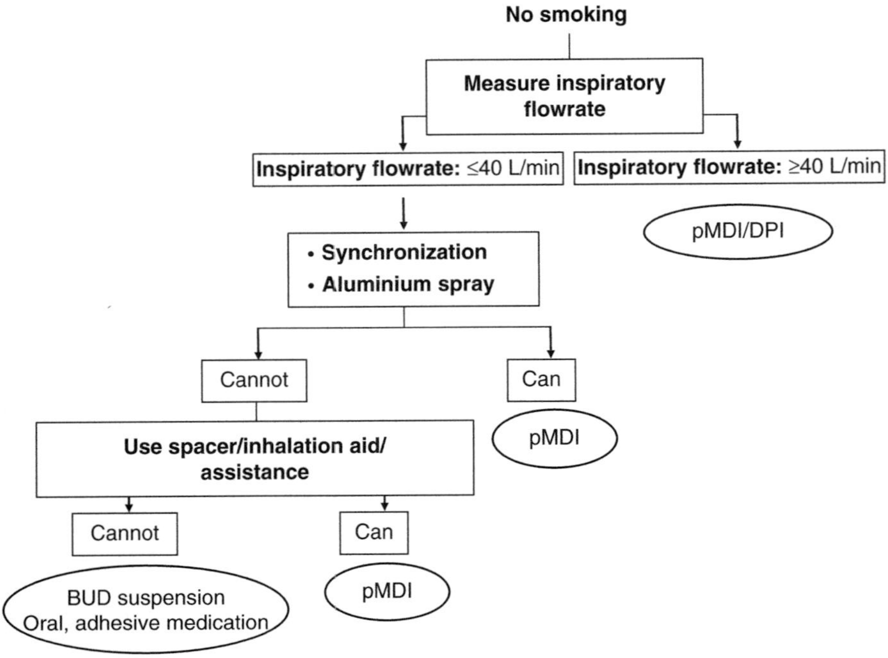

Fig. 12.2 Selection flowchart of pMDI and DPI for bronchial asthma

12.3 pMDI and DPI Selection Procedures

With the diversification of devices, doctors often hesitate over the criteria to use for selection. The authors have created a flow chart for pMDI and DPI selection procedures, based on inhalation flow rate, breath synchronization, and finger strength, and apply this flowchart in clinical practice (Fig. 12.2).

12.4 Techniques of Introducing a DVD for Inhalation Instructions

The authors created an inhalation instruction DVD in cooperation with the Environmental Restoration and Conservation Agency, aiming to ensure that patients will receive fixed instructions with as few omissions as possible, even when medical staff across Japan provide the inhalation instructions [9]. In 2015, we summarized the operating methods for all the different types of inhalants sold in Japan on an inhalation instruction DVD and poster entitled "Let's learn correct inhalation techniques," and these were made available for free-of-charge delivery throughout Japan (Fig. 12.3) (Inquiries: Environmental Restoration and Conservation Agency URL: http://www.erca.go.jp). Using this information enabled standardized inhalation instructions to be provided in a set period of time, and this learning was found to have a positive effect on outcomes, including pulmonary function [11]. The results were published in JGL,

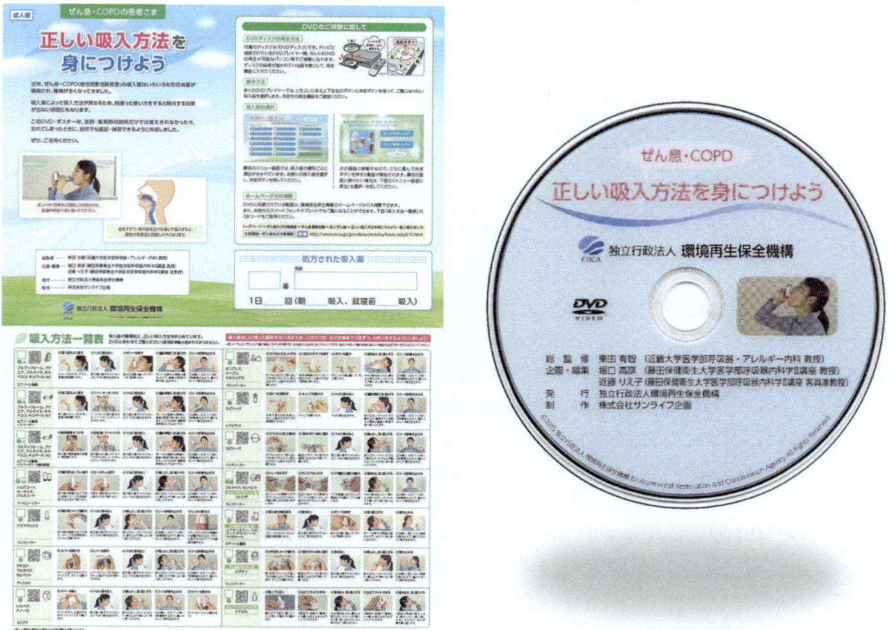

Fig. 12.3 DVD and poster entitled "Let's learn correct inhalation techniques"

2017 [2]. The DVD can be handed to individual patients, and they can watch it in their own homes. "Dealing with asthma attacks at home" is written on the back of the poster (bottom left), and it states the name of the drug to use for treating an attack, and when to use the drug, in an easy-to-understand format.

12.5 Key Points of Inhalation Instructions

We leave the explanation of inhalation procedures for each device to the respective pharmaceutical companies, but the common inhalation instructions are written below.

(a) Points for initial inhalation instructions

- Explain the necessity of inhalant steroids (they are the most effective at inhibiting airway inflammation and the most basic asthma medication used worldwide).
- Dispel resistance to steroids (the administered dose is approximately 1/10th of that of oral or injected steroids, so that there are minimal adverse reactions).
- Inform the patients of adverse reactions (ICS, hoarseness, oral candidiasis, etc.; LABA, palpitations, headache, finger trembling, etc.).
- If the patient is not able to understand the instructions (elderly, children, disabled persons, etc.), have a key person attend the explanation.
- Handing over a pamphlet only is inadequate as an explanation; therefore, explain the technique carefully using the actual drug or a tester.

- The first number of air shots is not uniform. Have the device set up by a pharmacist before giving it to the patient.
- Explain the number of air shots required if the device has not been used for some time.

(b) Common considerations for all devices

- Straighten the back and exhale sufficiently (with DPI devices, do not breathe onto the mouthpiece).
- With pMDIs, there is an intake of air; therefore, grasp the mouthpiece lightly with the teeth to create a gap.
- With DPIs and SMIs, fully cover the mouthpiece with the lips to ensure that no air can escape and ensure that the corners of the mouth do not open.
- With pMDIs and SMIs, inhale deeply and slowly with a normal breath.
- With DPIs, use a deep, sharp intake of breath.
- Remove the device from the mouth and hold the breath for approximately 5 s.
- Breathe out slowly through the nose.
- Gargle (three times in the mouth and three times in the back of the throat); if all patients use a uniform approach, confusion will be avoided.
- To prevent local adverse reactions in the mouth, it is recommended to drink water before use. It is also recommended to drink and eat after gargling.
- When gargling is not possible, such as during nighttime SMART therapy, drink water to rinse out the mouth and throat.
- If synchronizing the breath with a pMDI is difficult, a spacer should be purchased. In this case, also explain the method for cleaning the spacer.

(c) The main points of inhalation instructions from the second visit onward include the following:

- Check that the patient has not stopped or reduced the dose of their medication of their own accord.
- Check compliance with the number of inhalations.
- Ascertain the number of SMART therapies used.
- Check that the patient is using proper inhalation techniques. Ask if they have any questions (use the actual device or tester whenever possible).
- Record any mistakes or improvements in the patient's medical chart, and check on these thoroughly at the next appointment.
- Check that the patient is able to gargle and clean the device after use.
- Check for onset of adverse reactions.

The inhalation speed differs for pMDIs, SMIs, and DPIs; thus, it is easy to create confusion. It is vital to take precautions to avoid using the different devices together.

12.6 Investigating Preferred Tongue Position

Even if the patient uses the device correctly, the route from the inhalation port to the airways can be blocked with the tongue. We made a paper tube of the same size and shape as the mouthpiece of a pressurized metered-dose inhaler (pMDI, Flutiform), fixed an endoscope at the center of the paper tube with tape, and filmed the intraoral conditions in 9 healthy volunteers with and without tongue lowering from the actual position where the inhalants are ejected. In all volunteers, the percentages of the visible posterior pharyngeal wall area were significantly higher when the tongue was lowered than when it was not. Our second study verified that lowering the tongue keeps the inflow route to the trachea for inhalants wide open (Fig.12.4) [12]. Healthy volunteers ($n = 6$) used a placebo inhaler (Flutiform® tester, Relvar® tester), and the difference in the inflow volume of the drug into the airways with and without the tongue being lowered was imaged

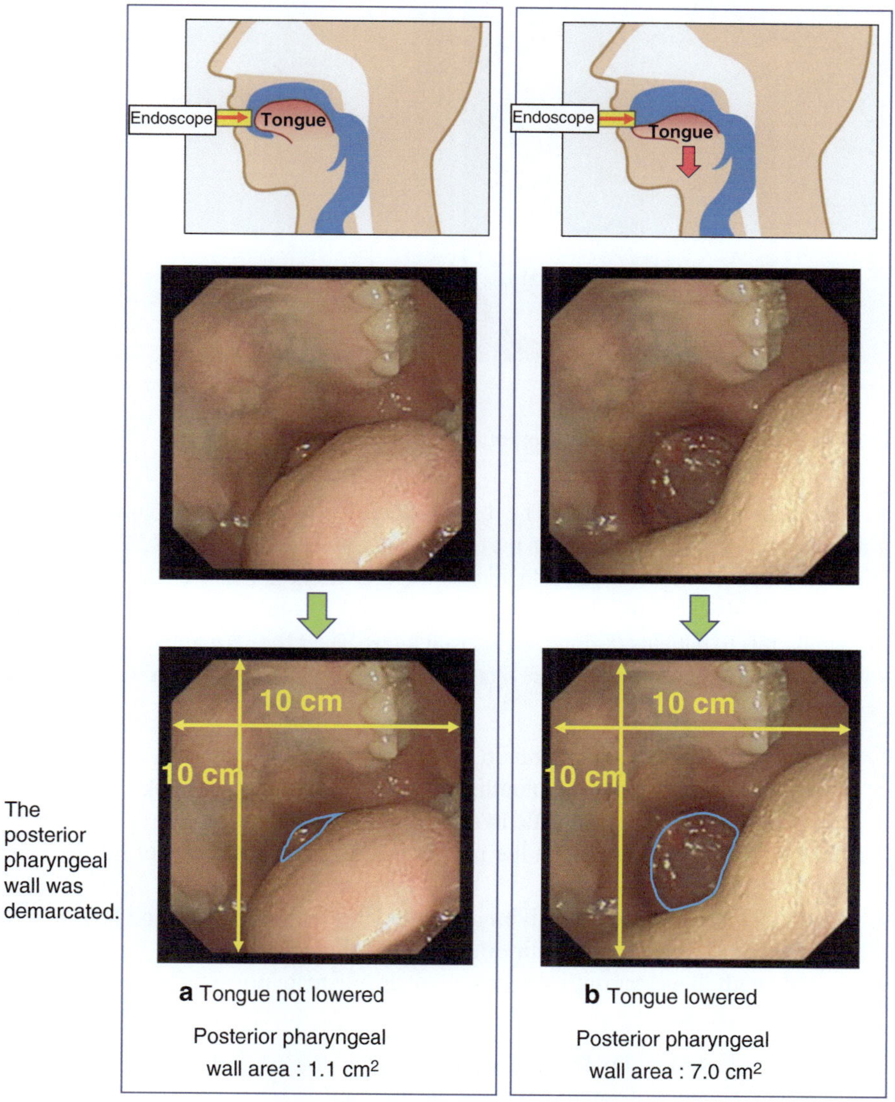

Fig. 12.4 Comparison of the area of posterior pharyngeal wall by tongue positions. (**a**) Tongue not lowered. Posterior pharyngeal wall area : 1.1 cm^2. (**b**) Tongue lowered. Posterior pharyngeal wall area: 7.0 cm^2. Yoshida T, et.al. J Allergy Clin Immunol Pract. 2018. https://doi.org/10.1016/j.jaip.2018.07.025

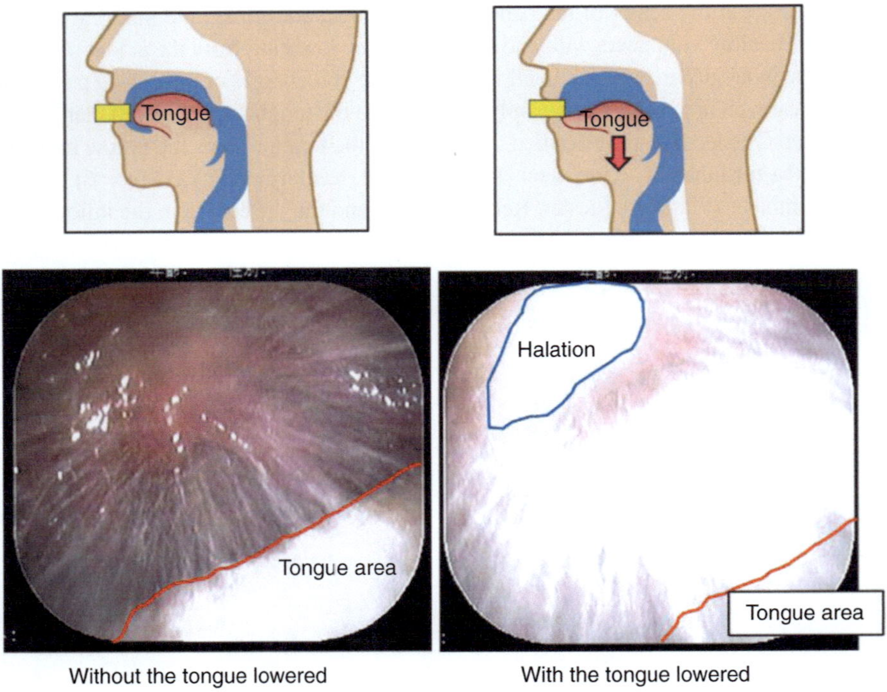

Fig. 12.5 Still image at maximum inflow of medication (Relvar® tester)

and analyzed with an endoscope. The results indicated that the inflow volume was significantly higher in all devices when the tongue was lowered [10] (Fig. 12.5). Therefore, inhaling with the tongue lowered facilitates more efficient delivery of the drug to the airways. This action cannot be checked visually, and it is difficult to allocate time to explaining this to patients during busy consultations. Therefore, the authors use the following method to explain and ensure that patients understand this concept within a short period of time [13].

1. Lift your face to ensure that you do not look down.
2. Place your tongue under the mouthpiece (if the tongue is not hooked under the tip of the mouthpiece, it is difficult to lower).
3. Make a "ho" sound, and form the image of a dome, like the spacer inside your mouth.
4. Once you have exhaled enough breath, think "ho!" in your mind and breath in.
5. Capture the feeling when the air directly hits the throat.
6. Practice with the tester until you can make an adequate noise (at a speed suitable for each device).

Then, show a patient DVD, hand the DVD to the patient, and ensure they master using the device, with the actual drug, in the pharmacy.

If the patient can understand the above instructions, the drug will reach the airways more reliably, thereby maximizing the therapeutic effect. This technique is the same for all inhalants.

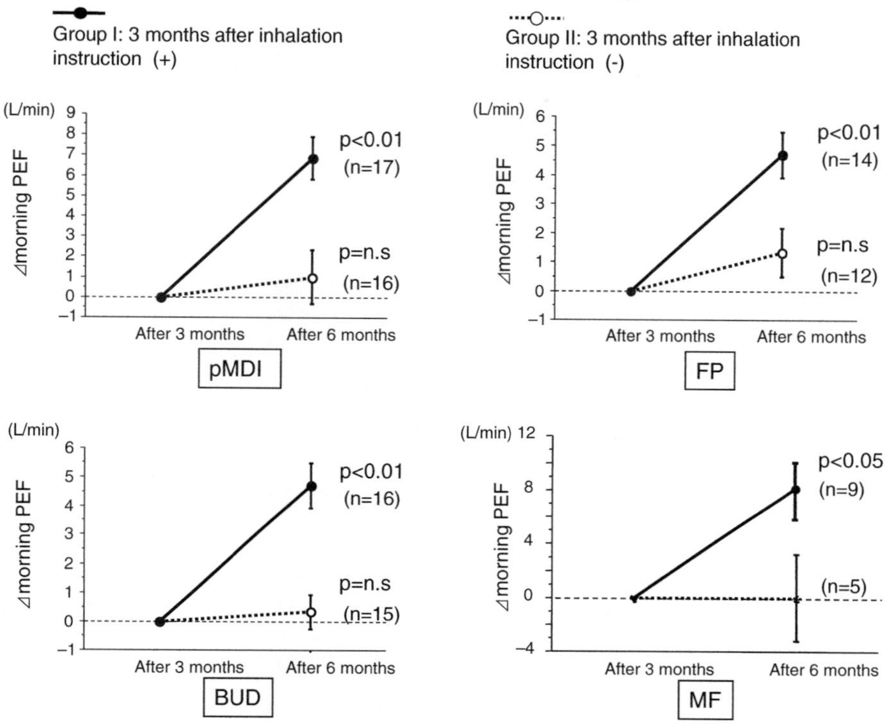

Fig. 12.6 Change in PEF after 6 months, with or without inhalation instruction (after 3 months)

12.7 Importance of Repeating Inhalation Instructions

A comparative study of peak expiratory flow was conducted in elderly patients, aged 65 years or older, with asthma. Two groups were provided inhalation instructions for each inhalant at the initial administration, and the inhalation instructions were repeated/checked after 3 months for one of the groups (Group I), while the other group did not receive the repeated instructions (Group II). Group I was significantly better at using all devices [14] (Fig. 12.6). Thus, it is important to repeat inhalation instructions.

12.8 Conclusion

Before stepping up the patient's treatment, it is vital to recheck the following. Is the drug/device suitable for the patient, given the patient's background? Is the drug being inhaled with the correct technique to ensure delivery to the airways? Irrespective of the age group, rechecking these points can prevent unnecessary step-up. It is important to make full use of tools, such as the inhalation instruction DVD, and it is important to repeat the inhalation instructions as long as the physician's time permits.

References

1. GINA guidelines. Global Initiative for asthma. 2016. www.ginasthma.org. Accessed 30 Oct 2017.
2. Asthma prevention and management guideline 2015 (JGL2015). Tokyo: Kyowa Kikaku; 2015.
3. Sanchis J, Gich I, Pedersen S. Aerosol drug management improvement team (ADMIT). Systematic review of errors in inhaler use: has patient technique improved over time? Chest. 2016;150(2):394–406.
4. Westerik JAM, Carter V, Chrystyn H, Burden A, Thompson SL, Ryan D, et al. Characteristics of patients making serious inhaler errors with a dry powder inhaler and association with asthma-related events in a primary care setting. J Asthma. 2016;53(3):321–9.
5. Price DB, Román-Rodríguez M, McQueen RB, Bosnic-Anticevich S, Carter V, Gruffydd-Jones K, et al. Inhaler errors in the CRITIKAL study: type, frequency, and association with asthma outcomes. J Allergy Clin Immunol Pract. 2017;5(4):1071–1081.e9.
6. Vrijens B, Dima AL, Van Ganse E, van Boven JF, Eakin MN, Foster JM, et al. What we mean when we talk about adherence in respiratory medicine. J Allergy Clin Immunol Pract. 2016;4(5):802–12.
7. Sulaiman I, Seheult J, MacHale E, D'Arcy S, Boland F, McCrory K, et al. Irregular and ineffective: a quantitative observational study of the time and technique of inhaler use. J Allergy Clin Immunol Pract. 2016;4(5):900–909.e2.
8. Press VG, Kelly CA, Kim JJ, White SR, Meltzer DO, Arora VM. Virtual Teach-To-Goal™ adaptive learning of inhaler technique for inpatients with asthma or COPD. J Allergy Clin Immunol Pract. 2017;5(4):1032–1039.e1.
9. Toda Y, Horiguchi T, Kondo R. Let's learn correct inhalation techniques. Kawasaki-Shi: Environmental Restoration and Conservation Agency; 2015.
10. Horiguchi T, Kondo R. Improving adherence. Med Pract. 2016;33(12):1973–8.
11. Takita K, Kondo K, Horiguchi T. Effectiveness of training patients using DVD in the accurate use of inhalers for the treatment of bronchial asthma. Allergol Int. 2017;66(4):545–9.
12. Yoshida T, Kondo R, Horiguchi T. A comparison of posterior pharyngeal wall areas between different tongue positions during inhalation. J Allergy Clin Immunol Pract. 2018.
13. Horiguchi T, Kondo R. Determination of the preferred tongue position for optimal inhaler use. J Allergy Clin Immunol Pract. 2018;6(3):1039–1041.e3.
14. Horiguchi T, Kondo R, et al. Treatment navigation in consideration of a characteristic of the elderly asthma. Allerg Immunol. 2010;17(6):108–15.

Chapter 13
Treatment with Anti-IgE Monoclonal Antibody and Free IgE

Hisako Matsumoto

Abstract Treatment with omalizumab, a monoclonal anti-IgE antibody, significantly reduces asthma symptoms, frequency of reliever use, and severe asthma exacerbations while improving pulmonary function in patients with severe allergic asthma who experience inadequate control with high doses of inhaled corticosteroids and other controllers. Airway tissue measurements and computed tomography have also shown that omalizumab treatment improves airway remodeling. In addition, omalizumab may augment protective effects against rhinovirus infection by potentially improving type I interferon production. Comorbidities related to severe asthma, such as eosinophilic chronic rhinosinusitis, allergic bronchopulmonary aspergillosis, and aspirin-exacerbated respiratory diseases, also respond to omalizumab treatment. Thus, omalizumab has introduced a new era for the management of severe asthma. However, given the heterogeneous nature of severe asthma, responses to omalizumab vary in patients with severe allergic asthma. Better responses to omalizumab are expected in patients with type 2-high inflammation who show higher levels of exhaled nitric oxide, blood eosinophils, and serum periostin. Lastly, the optimal duration of omalizumab treatment remains unknown, though discontinuation of omalizumab after a 5-year treatment period yielded significantly worse outcomes for asthma control than continuation thereof. Subsequently, higher blood eosinophil counts have been suggested to predict failure after treatment discontinuation.

Keywords Omalizumab · Type 2 inflammation · Free IgE

H. Matsumoto (✉)
Department of Respiratory Medicine, Kyoto University of Graduate School of Medicine, Kyoto University, Kyoto City, Kyoto, Japan
e-mail: hmatsumo@kuhp.kyoto-u.ac.jp

A. Yokoyama (ed.), *Advances in Asthma*, Respiratory Disease Series: Diagnostic Tools and Disease Managements, https://doi.org/10.1007/978-981-13-2790-2_13

13.1 Introduction

Omalizumab, a monoclonal anti-IgE antibody, is the first biologic therapy for patients with severe asthma. Omalizumab treatment has been known to significantly improve quality of life and pulmonary function while reducing asthma symptoms and frequency of severe asthma exacerbations in patients with severe allergic asthma. Nevertheless, not all patients respond equally to omalizumab treatment considering the heterogeneity of those with severe asthma. Therefore, biomarkers and clinical features of responders and incomplete responders should be elucidated for the efficient use of omalizumab in the management of severe asthma. Furthermore, questions regarding target patients and duration of omalizumab treatment still remain unresolved.

This chapter describes the mechanisms of action and effectiveness of omalizumab against severe allergic asthma and its comorbidities. In addition, biomarkers and patient characteristics that promote the optimal administration, monitoring, and safe discontinuation of omalizumab are highlighted.

13.2 Omalizumab Mechanisms of Action

13.2.1 Basic Mechanisms

Omalizumab is a humanized anti-IgE monoclonal antibody that specifically binds to the Cε3 region of the Fc fragment of IgE, thus inhibiting the binding between serum free IgE and high-affinity receptors (FcεRI) on mast cells, basophils, and dendritic cells and low-affinity receptors (FcεRII or CD23), which play a pivotal role in IgE homeostasis, on lymphocytes and eosinophils. Inhibiting the binding between free IgE and FcεRI prevents the release of various inflammatory mediators, such as histamine, leukotrienes, and prostaglandins, from mast cells (Fig. 13.1) [1]. However, omalizumab does not bind to IgE already bound to FcεRI on the membranes of mast cells or basophils and thus does not initiate allergic reactions.

In addition to its direct effects on "allergic reaction," omalizumab may be an essential disease modifier given its reduction of FcεRI expression and IgE production [2]. The airway tissues of omalizumab-treated patients exhibited a decrease in IgE-positive cells irrespective of their atopic status [3, 4]. Other studies showed that omalizumab treatment reduced the expression of FcεRI on mast cells and basophils [5]. Inhibiting the binding between free IgE and FcεRI on dendritic cells prevents the presentation of allergens from dendritic cells to Th2 cells, which in turn reduces IgE production by B cells (Fig. 13.1) [1]. Furthermore, one study revealed that omalizumab decreased IgE production in IL-4 and CD40 ligand-stimulated B cells [6], while another showed that omalizumab reduced IgE production in B cells via the reduction of germline Cε and IL-4R mRNA levels without affecting that of CD23 [7].

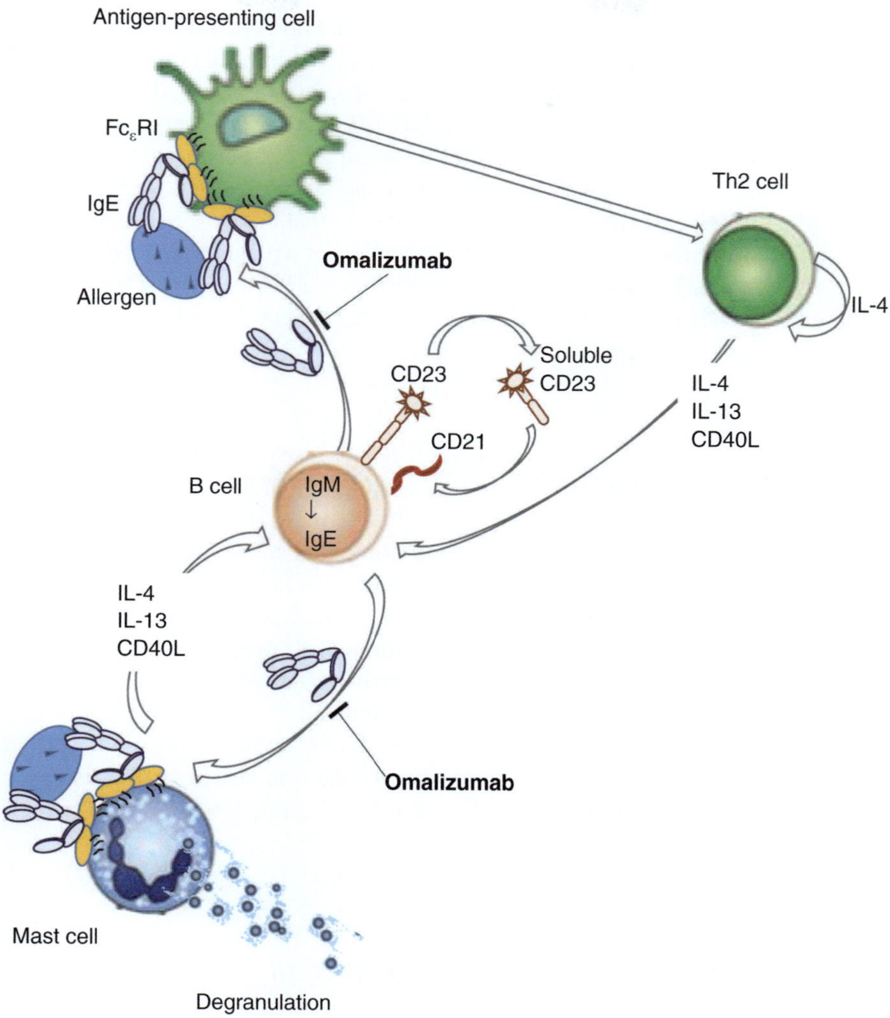

Fig. 13.1 Mechanisms of action of omalizumab, based on a review by Gould et al. [1]

13.3 Role of Omalizumab in Severe Allergic Asthma

13.3.1 General Effects

Omalizumab has been globally approved for the treatment of severe or moderate to severe allergic asthma in adults and children 12 years or older. Omalizumab is administered subcutaneously every 2 or 4 weeks at a dose determined according to the patient's body weight and serum total IgE levels (30–1500 IU/mL), ranging from 75 to 600 mg. Omalizumab exerts a number of effects [8], including improvement in quality of life and pulmonary function and reduction in asthma symptoms, asthma exacerbations, and doses of oral and inhaled corticosteroids. A meta-analysis of eight randomized controlled studies showed that omalizumab decreased severe asthma exacerbations by 43% [9]. A study conducted on an Asian population showed a significant increase in morning peak flow after 16 weeks of omalizumab treatment, as well as a 68% decrease in the frequency of clinically significant asthma exacerbations when compared to that before omalizumab treatment [10]. Moreover, using the Global Evaluation of Treatment Effectiveness, a meta-analysis of 25 real-world studies revealed that 77% of patients with severe asthma experienced remarkable or moderate improvement 4–6 months after starting omalizumab treatment [11].

13.3.2 Airway Remodeling

Direct measurement of airway tissues and computed tomography showed that omalizumab treatment improves airway remodeling. One year after omalizumab treatment, patients with severe allergic asthma experienced a reduction in airway basement layer thickening and eosinophil infiltrates accompanied by a reduction in the IgE-binding protein galectin-3 [12]. Omalizumab treatment also inhibited extracellular matrix production and collagen deposition of airway smooth muscle cells derived from atopic patients with moderate asthma. Moreover, studies using computed tomography showed an improvement in airway wall thickening among patients with severe asthma after 16 weeks [13] or 1 year of omalizumab treatment [14].

13.3.3 Potential Effects on IFN-α Production

Several studies have shown that the induction of type I interferon from airway epithelial cells or macrophages after rhinovirus infection, a major trigger of asthma exacerbation, is reduced in patients with asthma. In addition, in vitro studies have revealed the binding between IgE and FcεRI decreases the type I interferon production in plasma myelocytes. Recent studies on children with severe allergic asthma demonstrated that omalizumab may possibly augment protective effects against rhinovirus infection while improving the production of type I interferons by reducing the binding between IgE and FcεRI. Indeed, omalizumab treatment in children with severe asthma decreased asthma exacerbations in autumn, a peak season for asthma exacerbations and rhinovirus infections [15]. Moreover, blood monocytes produced greater amounts of type I interferons in children who responded to omalizumab treatment than in those who did not.

13.4 Biomarkers for Companion Diagnostics and Monitoring

13.4.1 Type 2 Markers

Although omalizumab has proven to be effective in patients with severe allergic asthma, patient responses to omalizumab have varied from excellent to mild. The EXTRA omalizumab study had reported on the utility of type 2 biomarkers using the reduction in asthma exacerbations during the first year of treatment to predict the efficacy of omalizumab. Accordingly, patients with higher levels of exhaled nitric oxide (FeNO), blood eosinophils, and serum periostin at baseline were more responsive to omalizumab treatment than those with lower levels thereof [16]. This was confirmed by Tajiri et al. who showed that higher FeNO levels were the best predictive marker of improvement in asthma control 16 weeks after treatment and that higher serum periostin levels were the best predictive marker of reduction in severe exacerbations 1 year after omalizumab treatment (Fig. 13.2) [17]. In addition, baseline serum periostin levels alone were negatively associated with free serum IgE levels after 16 or 32 weeks of treatment. A recent study that used patient enrichment criteria from omalizumab trials also confirmed that higher baseline blood eosinophil levels were related to greater reductions in exacerbation rates 16 weeks after omalizumab treatment [18].

13.4.2 Serum Total and Free IgE

As previously mentioned, long-term omalizumab treatment could possibly decrease B cell IgE production. Accordingly, Lowe and Renard established mathematical models for changes in serum total IgE levels, subsequently showing decreased IgE production

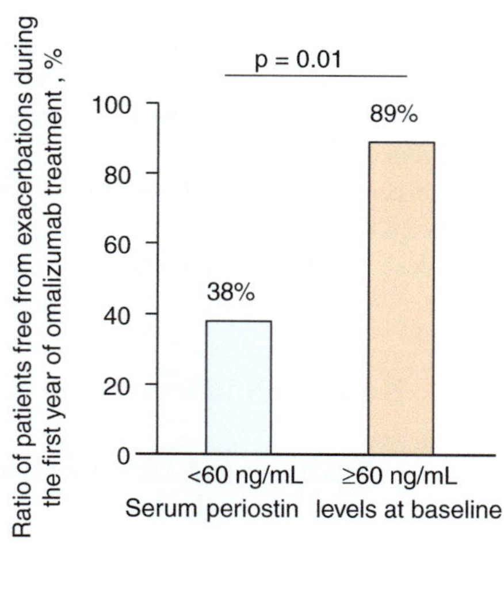

Fig. 13.2 The proportion of patients free from asthma exacerbations 1 year after omalizumab treatment stratified according to baseline serum periostin levels

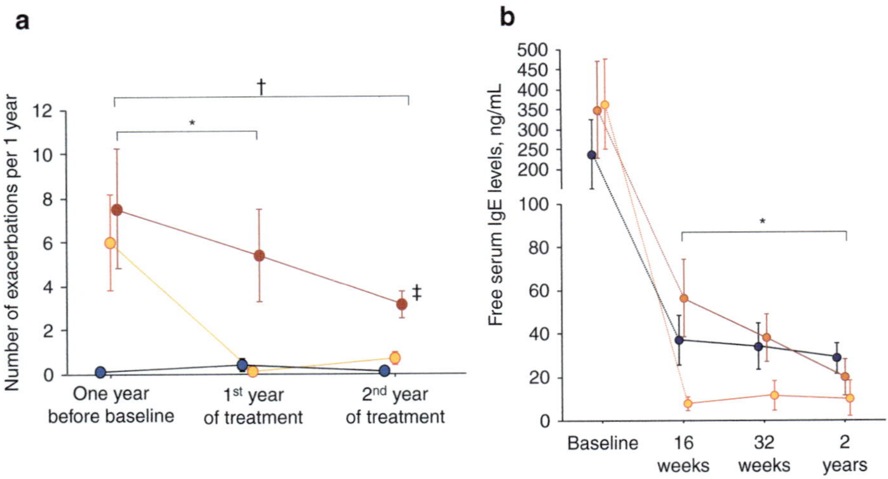

Fig. 13.3 (**a**) Frequencies of exacerbations and (**b**) serum free IgE levels monitored over 2 years of omalizumab treatment. The red circle indicates average serum free IgE levels of patients who still experienced asthma exacerbations during the first year of omalizumab treatment. The orange circle indicates average serum free IgE levels of patients who experienced asthma exacerbations 1 year before but not 1 year after omalizumab treatment. The blue circle indicates average serum free IgE levels of patients who did not experience asthma exacerbations both pre- and post-omalizumab treatment

in patients treated with omalizumab [2]. Thus, serum total IgE levels could be used for patient monitoring during omalizumab treatment. However, we need to consider that serum total IgE levels, which are the sum of free IgE and omalizumab-IgE complexes, increase temporarily after omalizumab administration given that the binding between omalizumab and free IgE extends the half-life of IgE from 2.4 to 20 days. Meanwhile, serum free IgE, a direct target of omalizumab, dramatically decreases following omalizumab initiation, subsequently reaching its target levels (<25–50 ng/mL) in most cases (Fig. 13.3) [19]. In addition, free IgE levels during treatment may be used to assess responsiveness to omalizumab treatment. Accordingly, Tajiri et al. showed that a decline in serum free IgE levels from baseline to 16 or 32 weeks after treatment was associated with reduced exacerbation frequency 2 years after omalizumab treatment [17]. Thus, serum free IgE levels can be useful for monitoring both short- and long-term omalizumab treatments [17, 20, 21]. Finally, physicians may opt to readjust omalizumab doses based on free IgE levels in stable patients after long-term omalizumab treatment.

13.5 Role of Omalizumab in Severe Asthma Comorbidities

13.5.1 Eosinophilic Chronic Rhinosinusitis (ECRS)

Eosinophilic chronic rhinosinusitis (ECRS), a subtype of chronic rhinosinusitis with eosinophil-enriched nasal polyps and often considered a synonym of chronic rhinosinusitis with nasal polyps (CRSwNP), is an intractable

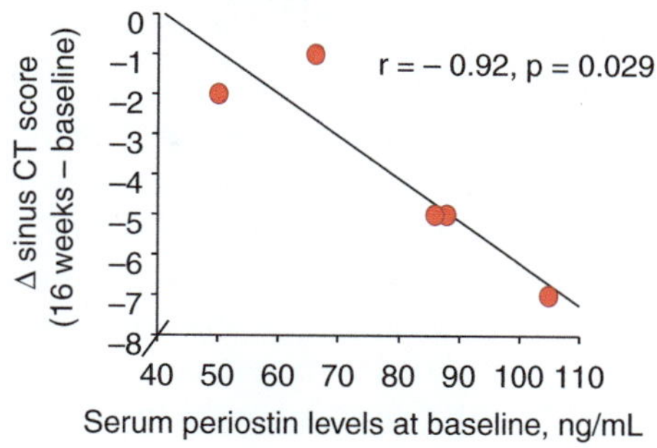

Fig. 13.4 Association between changes in sinus computed tomography scores and baseline serum periostin levels

comorbidity of severe asthma. Given that IgE levels, in particular against *Staphylococcus aureus* enterotoxin, are often elevated in nasal polyps of ECRS, the anti-IgE antibody omalizumab is expected to improve ECRS. A randomized, double-blind, placebo-controlled study of patients with nasal polyps and comorbid asthma ($n = 15$ for omalizumab vs. $n = 8$ for placebo) showed that 16 weeks of omalizumab treatment significantly improved nasal congestion and sense of smell and reduced nasal polyp sizes compared to placebo treatment [22]. In this study, patient recruitment had not been limited to those with severe asthma, while the efficacy of omalizumab had been reported in six patients with ECRS and severe asthma [23]. Consistent with the aforementioned study, total and rhinological symptom scores, including nasal blockage and dysosmia, sinus CT scores particularly in the ethmoid sinus, and sizes of nasal polyps were significantly improved 16 weeks after omalizumab treatment [23]. Such improvements were accompanied by improved asthma control scores and were correlated with changes in sputum eosinophil counts, closing volume, and serum periostin levels and with baseline serum periostin levels (Fig. 13.4). These associations suggest that omalizumab may be effective against the comorbidity between ECRS and severe allergic asthma.

13.5.2 Aspirin-Exacerbated Respiratory Disease (AERD)

AERD is a subtype of severe asthma that is characterized by a triad of asthma, ECRS, and intolerance to nonsteroidal anti-inflammatory drugs. The basic feature of AERD includes explosive constriction of both upper and lower airways triggered by the use of cyclooxygenase-1 inhibitors. Mast cell activation may be involved in the pathobiology of AERD given the overproduction of leukotriene E_4. Hayashi et al. revealed that omalizumab treatment reduced daily oral corticosteroid doses and frequency of asthma exacerbations in patients with AERD [24], among whom 18/21 (85.7%) were overall responders. After omalizumab treatment, urinary concentrations of leukotriene E_4 and prostaglandin D_2 metabolite 9α,11β-prostaglandin F_2 significantly decreased by 76.2% and 89.0%, respectively. These improvements may be attributed to the stabilization of mast cell activity after omalizumab treatment.

13.5.3 Allergic Bronchopulmonary Aspergillosis (ABPA)

ABPA is an allergic disease that is characterized by severe asthma, recurrent and transient pulmonary infiltrates, blood eosinophilia, central bronchiectasis, and elevated serum total and *Aspergillus fumigatus*-specific IgE levels and *Aspergillus fumigatus*-specific IgG levels. Accordingly, Tillie-Leblond et al. demonstrated that patients with ABPA (n = 16) had significantly fewer asthma exacerbations and lower doses of oral corticosteroids 1 year after than 1 year before omalizumab treatment [25]. Moreover, a prospective study by Voskamp et al. showed that patients with ABPA (n = 13) exhibited a significant reduction in asthma exacerbations, exhaled nitric oxide levels, and expression of FcεRI on basophils after omalizumab treatment [26]. Thus, based on the aforementioned studies, omalizumab may be effective against ABPA.

13.5.4 Asthma-COPD Overlap (ACO)

Despite the absence of an established definition, the term ACO encompasses several different phenotypes. Nonetheless, a promising finding by Maltby et al. suggested that patients suffering from severe allergic asthma and physician-diagnosed COPD showed significant improvements in asthma control and health-related quality of life [27]. In such patients, however, lung function and the activity component of the Asthma Quality of Life Questionnaire score did not improve after omalizumab treatment.

13.5.5 Chronic Idiopathic Urticaria

Mast cell activation is an important feature of urticaria. In severe cases of chronic idiopathic urticaria, mast cell activation becomes resistant to antihistamine medications. Omalizumab has proven to be effective against chronic idiopathic urticaria, demonstrating apparent reductions in itch scores within 12 weeks. Currently, omalizumab is prescribed to patients with chronic idiopathic urticaria regardless of the presence of severe asthma.

13.6 Incomplete Responders to Omalizubmab

As previously mentioned, ECRS and AERD are typical type 2 inflammatory diseases that are responsive to omalizumab treatment. However, some ECRS and AERD cases may exhibit incomplete responses to omalizumab treatment. A real-world study revealed that patients with comorbidities, such as CRSwNP, AERD, gastroesophageal reflux disease, and obesity, displayed poorer asthma control after omalizumab treatment than those without the same [28].

Although some atopic patients with early-onset asthma do not show prominent eosinophilic/type 2 inflammation, they slowly respond to omalizumab treatment. Tajiri et al. showed that patients who had severe asthma exacerbations 1 year after omalizumab treatment were relatively younger at asthma onset and were atopic despite having lower blood eosinophil counts at baseline [17]. However, in those patients with low blood eosinophil counts, the frequency of severe asthma exacerbations significantly decreased together with the gradual decrease in serum free IgE levels after a 2-year follow-up (Fig. 13.3). Although responses to omalizumab were slow and incomplete, omalizumab may be an important medication for patients with early-onset atopic asthma, but not prominent eosinophilic/type 2 inflammation. Theoretically, such patients may not benefit much from anti-IL-5 biologics.

13.7 Long-Term Use of Omalizumab and Possibility of Discontinuation

13.7.1 Efficacy of Long-Term Omalizumab Use

Omalizumab had been first approved in Australia (2002) followed by the United States (2003), the European Union (2005), and Japan (2009). Thus, sufficient evidence on the long-term use of omalizumab treatment has been accumulated. One study examined the efficacy of omalizumab according to the length of treatment period and found no significant differences in the status of asthma control after 4–6, 12, and 24 months of treatment. This study concluded that the efficacy of omalizumab did not attenuate even after long-term treatment. Sposato et al. showed that among patients receiving omalizumab treatment, those treated for 5 years or longer were able to significantly step down their asthma medications compared to those having shorter treatment periods [29]. Moreover, among several asthma medications, long-acting beta agonists, montelukast, and oral corticosteroids were significantly reduced during treatment step-down.

13.7.2 Possibility of Omalizumab Treatment Discontinuation

An earlier study involving omalizumab discontinuation after 28 weeks of treatment showed that asthma symptoms re-emerged and suppressed free IgE levels returned to baseline within 18–20 weeks [19]. Thus, 28 weeks of treatment may be insufficient to fully benefit from omalizumab treatment. Moreover, among 61 patients who discontinued omalizumab treatment after an average duration of 22.7 ± 13.1 months, 55.7% developed loss of asthma control within a median interval of 13 months [30].

One study reported successful discontinuation of omalizumab in 12 of 18 patients after 5–6 years of treatment [31], while another noted discontinuation failure in 9 of 11 patients [32]. Although identifying factors that lead to discontinuation failure may prove to be difficult, one such factor may include the presence of severe asthma exacerbations 1 year prior to discontinuation. Ledford et al. conducted a prospective study on persistency of omalizumab response after long-term omalizumab treatment (n = 176). Accordingly, 72.9% of patients who continued omalizumab treatment were free from asthma exacerbations during the following year, whereas only 53.5% of patients who discontinued omalizumab treatment experienced the same [33]. Asthma control test scores were also significantly better in patients who continued omalizumab treatment than in those who did not. Among patients who discontinued treatment, those who experienced asthma exacerbations showed higher blood eosinophil counts than those who were free from exacerbations. These findings may suggest that the presence of severe type 2 inflammation may hinder the successful discontinuation of omalizumab treatment.

13.8 Conclusion

Omalizumab has introduced a paradigm shift in the management of severe asthma. Although target patients of omalizumab overlap with those of several other anti-type 2 biologics that are available currently or in the near future, the unique aspects of omalizumab, such as disease modification and mast cell deactivation, should be emphasized. Accordingly, further studies are needed to elucidate the target patients and optimal treatment duration of omalizumab.

References

1. Gould HJ, Sutton BJ. IgE in allergy and asthma today. Nat Rev Immunol. 2008;8:205–17.
2. Lowe PJ, Renard D. Omalizumab decreases IgE production in patients with allergic (IgE-mediated) asthma; PKPD analysis of a biomarker, total IgE. Br J Clin Pharmacol. 2011;72:306–20.
3. Djukanovic R, Wilson SJ, Kraft M, Jarjour NN, Steel M, Chung KF, et al. Effects of treatment with anti-immunoglobulin E antibody omalizumab on airway inflammation in allergic asthma. Am J Respir Crit Care Med. 2004;170:583–93.
4. Pillai P, Chan YC, Wu SY, Ohm-Laursen L, Thomas C, Durham SR, et al. Omalizumab reduces bronchial mucosal IgE and improves lung function in non-atopic asthma. Eur Respir J. 2016;48:1593–601.
5. Beck LA, Marcotte GV, MacGlashan D, Togias A, Saini S. Omalizumab-induced reductions in mast cell Fce psilon RI expression and function. J Allergy Clin Immunol. 2004;114:527–30.
6. Hanf G, Brachmann I, Kleine-Tebbe J, Seybold J, Kunkel G, Suttorp N, et al. Omalizumab decreased IgE-release and induced changes in cellular immunity in patients with allergic asthma. Allergy. 2006;61:1141–4.

7. Chan MA, Gigliotti NM, Dotson AL, Rosenwasser LJ. Omalizumab may decrease IgE synthesis by targeting membrane IgE+ human B cells. Clin Transl Allergy. 2013;3:29.
8. Busse W, Corren J, Lanier BQ, McAlary M, Fowler-Taylor A, Cioppa GD, et al. Omalizumab, anti-IgE recombinant humanized monoclonal antibody, for the treatment of severe allergic asthma. J Allergy Clin Immunol. 2001;108:184–90.
9. Rodrigo GJ, Neffen H, Castro-Rodriguez JA. Efficacy and safety of subcutaneous omalizumab vs placebo as add-on therapy to corticosteroids for children and adults with asthma: a systematic review. Chest. 2011;139:28–35.
10. Ohta K, Miyamoto T, Amagasaki T, Yamamoto M. Efficacy and safety of omalizumab in an Asian population with moderate-to-severe persistent asthma. Respirology. 2009;14:1156–65.
11. Alhossan A, Lee CS, MacDonald K, Abraham I. "Real-life" effectiveness studies of omalizumab in adult patients with severe allergic asthma: meta-analysis. J Allergy Clin Immunol Pract. 2017;5:1362–70.e2.
12. Mauri P, Riccio AM, Rossi R, Di Silvestre D, Benazzi L, De Ferrari L, et al. Proteomics of bronchial biopsies: galectin-3 as a predictive biomarker of airway remodelling modulation in omalizumab-treated severe asthma patients. Immunol Lett. 2014;162:2–10.
13. Hoshino M, Ohtawa J. Effects of adding omalizumab, an anti-immunoglobulin E antibody, on airway wall thickening in asthma. Respiration. 2011;83:520–8.
14. Tajiri T, Niimi A, Matsumoto H, Ito I, Oguma T, Otsuka K, et al. Comprehensive efficacy of omalizumab for severe refractory asthma: a time-series observational study. Ann Allergy Asthma Immunol. 2014;113:470–5.e2.
15. Teach SJ, Gill MA, Togias A, Sorkness CA, Arbes SJ Jr, Calatroni A, et al. Preseasonal treatment with either omalizumab or an inhaled corticosteroid boost to prevent fall asthma exacerbations. J Allergy Clin Immunol. 2015;136:1476–85.
16. Hanania NA, Wenzel S, Rosen K, Hsieh HJ, Mosesova S, Choy DF, et al. Exploring the effects of omalizumab in allergic asthma: an analysis of biomarkers in the EXTRA study. Am J Respir Crit Care Med. 2013;187:804–11.
17. Tajiri T, Matsumoto H, Gon Y, Ito R, Hashimoto S, Izuhara K, et al. Utility of serum periostin and free IgE levels in evaluating responsiveness to omalizumab in patients with severe asthma. Allergy. 2016;71(10):1472–9.
18. Casale TB, Chipps BE, Rosen K, Trzaskoma B, Haselkorn T, Omachi TA, et al. Response to omalizumab using patient enrichment criteria from trials of novel biologics in asthma. Allergy. 2017;73:490–7.
19. Slavin RG, Ferioli C, Tannenbaum SJ, Martin C, Blogg M, Lowe PJ. Asthma symptom re-emergence after omalizumab withdrawal correlates well with increasing IgE and decreasing pharmacokinetic concentrations. J Allergy Clin Immunol. 2009;123:107–13.e3.
20. Ito R, Gon Y, Nunomura S, Atsuta R, Harada N, Hattori T, et al. Development of assay for determining free IgE levels in serum from patients treated with omalizumab. Allergol Int. 2014;63(Suppl 1):37–47.
21. Gon Y, Ito R, Maruoka S, Mizumura K, Kozu Y, Hiranuma H, et al. Long-term course of serum total and free IgE levels in severe asthma patients treated with omalizumab. Allergol Int. 2018;67(2):283–5.
22. Gevaert P, Calus L, Van Zele T, Blomme K, De Ruyck N, Bauters W, et al. Omalizumab is effective in allergic and nonallergic patients with nasal polyps and asthma. J Allergy Clin Immunol. 2013;131:110–6.e1.
23. Tajiri T, Matsumoto H, Hiraumi H, Ikeda H, Morita K, Izuhara K, et al. Efficacy of omalizumab in eosinophilic chronic rhinosinusitis patients with asthma. Ann Allergy Asthma Immunol. 2013;110:387–8.
24. Hayashi H, Mitsui C, Nakatani E, Fukutomi Y, Kajiwara K, Watai K, et al. Omalizumab reduces cysteinyl leukotriene and 9alpha,11beta-prostaglandin F2 overproduction in aspirin-exacerbated respiratory disease. J Allergy Clin Immunol. 2015;137:1585–7.e4.
25. Tillie-Leblond I, Germaud P, Leroyer C, Tetu L, Girard F, Devouassoux G, et al. Allergic bronchopulmonary aspergillosis and omalizumab. Allergy. 2011;66:1254–6.

26. Voskamp AL, Gillman A, Symons K, Sandrini A, Rolland JM, O'Hehir RE, et al. Clinical efficacy and immunologic effects of omalizumab in allergic bronchopulmonary aspergillosis. J Allergy Clin Immunol Pract. 2015;3:192–9.
27. Maltby S, Gibson PG, Powell H, McDonald VM. Omalizumab treatment response in a population with severe allergic asthma and overlapping COPD. Chest. 2017;151:78–89.
28. Novelli F, Latorre M, Vergura L, Caiaffa MF, Camiciottoli G, Guarnieri G, et al. Asthma control in severe asthmatics under treatment with omalizumab: a cross-sectional observational study in Italy. Pulm Pharmacol Ther. 2015;31:123–9.
29. Sposato B, Scalese M, Latorre M, Novelli F, Scichilone N, Milanese M, et al. Can the response to Omalizumab be influenced by treatment duration? A real-life study. Pulm Pharmacol Ther. 2017;44:38–45.
30. Molimard M, Mala L, Bourdeix I, Le Gros V. Observational study in severe asthmatic patients after discontinuation of omalizumab for good asthma control. Respir Med. 2014;108:571–6.
31. Nopp A, Johansson SG, Adedoyin J, Ankerst J, Palmqvist M, Oman H. After 6 years with Xolair; a 3-year withdrawal follow-up. Allergy. 2010;65:56–60.
32. Kuprys-Lipinska I, Kuna P. Loss of asthma control after cessation of omalizumab treatment: real life data. Postepy Dermatol Alergol. 2014;31:1–5.
33. Ledford D, Busse W, Trzaskoma B, Omachi TA, Rosen K, Chipps BE, et al. A randomized multicenter study evaluating Xolair persistence of response after long-term therapy. J Allergy Clin Immunol. 2017;140:162–9.e2.

Chapter 14
Bronchial Thermoplasty: Japanese Experiences

Takashi Iwanaga, Akiko Sano, Osamu Nishiyama, Hiroyuki Sano, and Yuji Tohda

Abstract In the approximately 5–10% of asthma patients whose condition is poorly controlled, asthma is present even if the patient is treated with high-dose inhalational steroids and long-acting beta 2 agonists. We cauterized a bronchus of 3–10 mm inner diameter at 65 °C for patients with such severe asthma. Bronchial thermoplasty, which reduces the quantity of the airway smooth muscle, was introduced as an epoch-making treatment in Japan from 2015. Airway contraction is reduced through the reduction of the quantity of smooth muscle in the airway, and the palliation of symptoms is obtained. The efficacy and safety of bronchial thermoplasty is currently being examined by a multicenter study in Japan.

Keywords Asthma · Severe asthma · Bronchial thermoplasty · Airway smooth muscle

14.1 Introduction

In daily clinical practice related to asthma, the control of asthma has been improved by the spread of inhaled corticosteroids (ICS) and combination treatment with long-acting beta 2 agonists (LABAs) (ICS/LABA), and the number of asthma-related deaths decreased from 6370 patients in 1980 to 1454 in 2016. However, it is said that 5–10% of asthma patients often experience exacerbations of their symptoms, which cannot be controlled without the use of high-dose ICS/LABA [1]. In recent years,

T. Iwanaga (✉) · A. Sano · O. Nishiyama · H. Sano · Y. Tohda
Department of Respiratory Medicine and Allergology, Kindai University Faculty of Medicine, Osaka, Japan
e-mail: iwanga@med.kindai.ac.jp

A. Yokoyama (ed.), *Advances in Asthma*, Respiratory Disease Series: Diagnostic Tools and Disease Managements, https://doi.org/10.1007/978-981-13-2790-2_14

biological agents (anti-IgE, anti-IL-5, anti-IL-5Rα) have been introduced for the treatment of such patients; however, bronchial thermoplasty (BT), an epoch-making intervention in which the airway wall is heated, was introduced in Japan in 2015.

14.2 The History of Bronchial Thermoplasty Prior to its Clinical Application

Studies using animal models to investigate the effects of cauterizing the asthmatic airway using radiofrequency waves in order to reduce the quantity of airway smooth muscle began from early 2000. The initial studies were based on the results of the application of cauterization in the treatment of heart disease and malignant tumors. The cauterization of the airway led to a reduction of the airway smooth muscle and reduced airway hypersensitivity; these effects were maintained for 3 years [2]. The first report on human clinical trials was published in 2005 [3], and BT subsequently passed through a randomized trial for severe asthma before being authorized by the American Food and Drug Administration (FDA) in 2010. BT was introduced into Japan in 2015 and received insurance approval in April of that year.

14.3 The Significance of Bronchial Thermoplasty

The airway smooth muscle hyperplasia that results from chronic airway inflammation contributes to airflow limitations in asthma patients and causes airway contraction at the exacerbation of asthma and a worsening of symptoms. BT heats the airway wall with a radiofrequency wave of 65 °C for 10 s and reduces airway contraction by reducing the quantity of the airway smooth muscle, leading to the relief of asthma symptoms.

14.4 Indications and Contraindications of Bronchial Thermoplasty

The indications of BT include the presence of severe asthma in an asthma patient of ≥18 years of age, whose asthma symptoms cannot be controlled with high-dose ICS and LABA, in whom bronchoscopy is possible. A respirology or allergology specialist with sufficient knowledge and experience about the treatment of asthma in the clinical setting must decide the indications of BT. The BT procedure is performed under the instruction of a bronchoscopy specialist in the institution who can treat complications associated with the procedure. It is also necessary for the practiced hand to attend the training provided by the instrument manufacturer (Boston Scientific, Tokyo, Japan) beforehand.

BT is contraindicated for patients who cannot discontinue antithrombotic drugs, aspirin, NSAIDs, patients with implanted electrical devices, patients who require drugs for the performance of bronchoscopy, patients who have previously undergone BT in the same location, patients with respiratory infection, patients in whom the dose of oral corticosteroids is changed (increased or decreased) or who have experienced an asthma exacerbation in the past 14 days, and patients with suspected blood coagulation disorder. Furthermore, the indications for BT should be carefully considered for patients whose FEV_1 after the administration of bronchodilator is <65% of the predicted value, patients who require oral corticosteroids at a dose of >10 mg/day, patients who have required intubation due to an asthma exacerbation, patients who have been admitted to an intensive care unit (ICU) in the past 2 years, patients who have been admitted more than three times in the past year, patients who have experienced lower respiratory tract infections more than four times in the past year, and patients who require burst treatment with oral corticosteroids more than four times a year.

14.5 The Methods of Bronchial Thermoplasty

14.5.1 Three Days Before Procedure

One condition enforced for BT is that the patient does not experience an asthma exacerbation or a change in the conventional dose of oral corticosteroids within 2 weeks of the procedure day. The patients are given prednisolone (50 mg/day) for 5 days from 3 days before the procedure in order to prevent the exacerbation of airway inflammation.

14.5.2 The Day Before Undergoing the Procedure

The patient is admitted on the day before procedure and a blood test, chest X-ray, chest CT, and electrocardiography are performed to investigate the stability of their asthma.

14.5.3 The Day of the Procedure

At first a pulmonary function test is performed on the day of the procedure; it is confirmed that the FEV_1 after SABA is >85% of the normal values. SABA is then inhaled, and atropine is subsequently administered to inhibit respiratory secretion during the procedure. The procedure is performed under intravenous anesthesia or general anesthesia (we choose intravenous anesthesia in our department) because of the long procedure time (approximately 1 h).

14.5.4 *Instruments (Alair™ Bronchial Thermoplasty System Figs. 14.1, 14.2, and 14.3)*

An insulated flexible bronchoscope with an outer diameter of ≤5.3 mm and a channel diameter of ≥2 mm is used. The instrument is composed of an exclusive basket-type electrode catheter and controller and the counter electrode.

14.5.5 *The Regimen and Schedule*

The BT procedure is performed by three staff members: one operates the bronchoscope, one manipulates the catheter, and the other performs bronchial mapping and records the number of activations. The operator inserts a catheter in a bronchus with an inside diameter of 3 mm, and the catheter manipulator opens the basket and

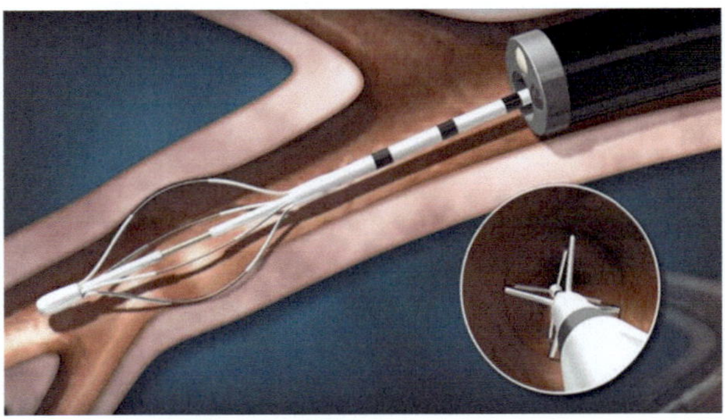

Fig. 14.1 Activation by electrode catheter (Permitted reprint by Boston Scientific)

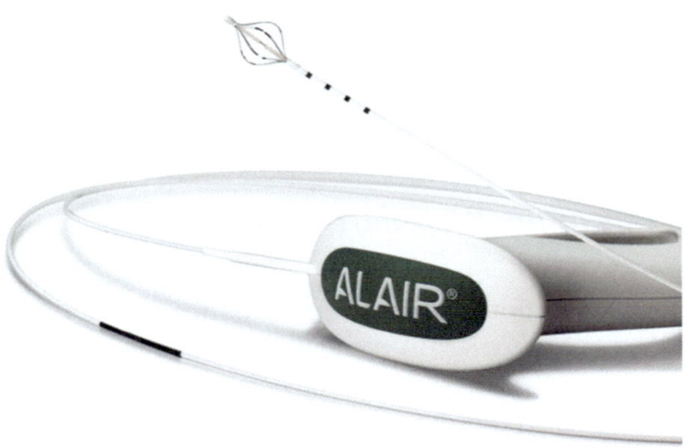

Fig. 14.2 Electrode catheter (Permitted reprint by Boston Scientific)

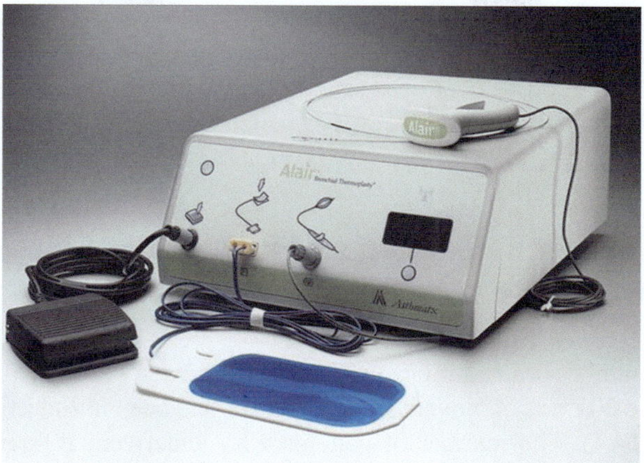

Fig. 14.3 Controller and counter electrode (Permitted reprint by Boston Scientific)

applies electricity for 10 s. The catheter is returned to the central side in 5 mm increments, and the application of electricity is repeated for a bronchus with an inside diameter of 10 mm. BT is scheduled to start at the right lower lobe, followed by left lower lobe, and both upper lobes, with a 3-week interval between the treatment of each lobe (in order to avoid the risk of the middle lobe syndrome, the middle lobe is not treated).

14.5.6 After the Procedure

A blood test, chest X-ray, and pulmonary function test are performed on the day after BT. Similarly before the procedure, the FEV_1 is confirmed to be >80%, and the patient does not have an exacerbation of asthma. The patient can be discharged after these points are confirmed. One week later, the patient is examined in an outpatient clinic, where a blood test, chest X-ray, and pulmonary function test are performed; the recovery of their pulmonary function and the presence or absence of complications are confirmed.

14.6 The Efficacy of Bronchial Thermoplasty (Abroad)

The randomized trials that led to the authorization of BT by the FDA include AIR (Asthma Intervention Research) [4], RISA (Research in Severe Asthma) [5], and AIR2 (Asthma Intervention Research 2) [6]. In the AIR trial, a reduction of moderate asthma exacerbations and asymptomatic days and improved asthma control and quality of life were observed in 55 patients with moderate-to-severe asthma after a year of BT [4]. In the RISA trial, short-acting beta 2 agonist usage, asthma control, quality of life, and the pulmonary function were improved at 22 weeks after BT in 15 patients with severe asthma [5]. The AIR2 trial, which was a double-blind sham study showed the improvement of severe asthma exacerbations, emergency visits, and quality of life at 1 year after BT in 190 patients with severe asthma [6].

14.7 The Present Conditions and Efficacy of Bronchial Thermoplasty in Japan

In Japan, the number of institutions in which BT has been introduced has gradually increased since 2015; as of November 1, 2017, BT had been introduced in 107 institutions (Fig. 14.4). The number of patients who underwent BT reached 450 on November 1, 2017 (Fig. 14.5). The characteristics of the cases were as follows: mean age, 53.8 ± 14.1 years; female, $n = 165$; male, $n = 260$; and mean FEV_1 (%predicted), 78.2 ± 20.3%. The mean number of activations and time required for treatment are shown in Table 14.1 (supplied by Boston Scientific).

A single-institution study of BT for Japanese asthma patients has been reported [7]. The characteristics of the 12 patients with severe asthma were as follows: mean age 56.1 ± 14.5 years; female, $n = 6$; male, $n = 6$; GINA treatment step 4, $n = 3$; and

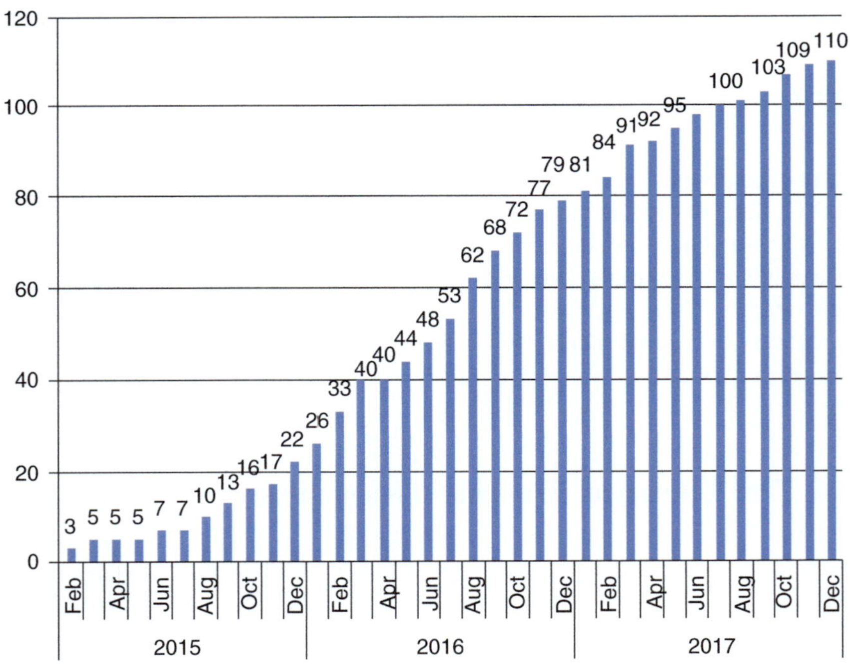

Fig. 14.4 Institutions introduced bronchial thermoplasty in Japan (accumulation, 1 January 2018) (Permitted reprint by Boston Scientific)

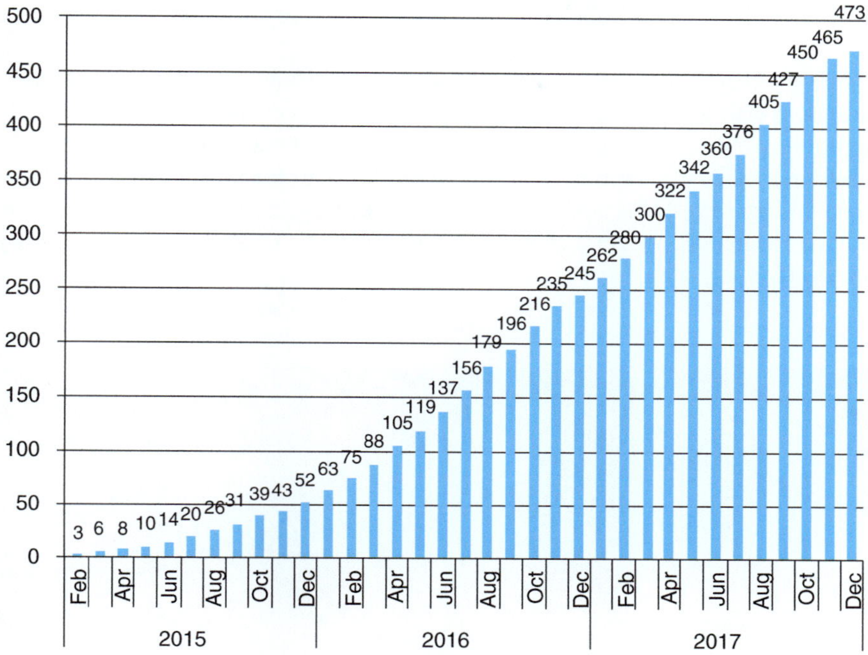

Fig. 14.5 Patients underwent bronchial thermoplasty in Japan (accumulation, 1 January 2018) (Permitted reprint by Boston Scientific)

Table 14.1 The mean number of activations and the time required for treatment of the bronchial thermoplasty in Japan ($n = 276$) (Permitted reprint by Boston Scientific)

Treatment times	Treatment area	Number of activation (mean ± SD)	Required time (min) (mean ± SD)
First	Right lower lobe	49.4 ± 17.9	43.1 ± 18.0
Second	Left lower lobe	48.4 ± 16.3	41.0 ± 16.0
Third	Right and left upper lobe	74.7 ± 24.4	53.8 ± 19.5

GINA treatment step 5, $n = 9$. The efficacy of BT was assessed at 1 year after BT according to the QOL (asthma-related quality of life questionnaire [AQLQ]), asthmatic control (asthma control questionnaire [ACQ-5], asthma control test [ACT]), the pulmonary function (FEV_1, %predicted), FeNO, the annual numbers of exacerbations and hospitalizations, and the degree of the treatment. The results that showed significant improvement were as follows: AQLQ (baseline, 4.9 ± 1.1; 1 year, 5.8 ± 1.3, $p < 0.05$), ACQ-5 (baseline, 1.5 ± 0.9; 1 year, 0.9 ± 0.9, $p < 0.05$), FEV1 (%predicted) (baseline, 70.5 ± 21.7; 1 year, 82.3 ± 21.8, $p < 0.01$), and annual number of exacerbations (baseline, 5.8 ± 5.3; 1 year, 2.0 ± 2.8, $p < 0.05$). The FeNO (ppb) (baseline, 50.2 ± 70.8; 1 year, 68.8 ± 21.8) did not show a significant improvement. It was suggested that BT did not show effect eosinophilic airway inflammation.

14.8 The Safety of BT [8]

The respiratory complications of BT include cough, sputum, wheezing, and shortness of breath and appear within 1 day after treatment; however, these usually improved within approximately 1 week with standard therapy. A chest X-ray shows infiltrative shadow at the treatment site on the day after treatment (Fig. 14.6); however, this improves after approximately 1 week. Atelectasis of the treatment site may be found, and attention should be paid to detect a decrease in the pulmonary function in such cases.

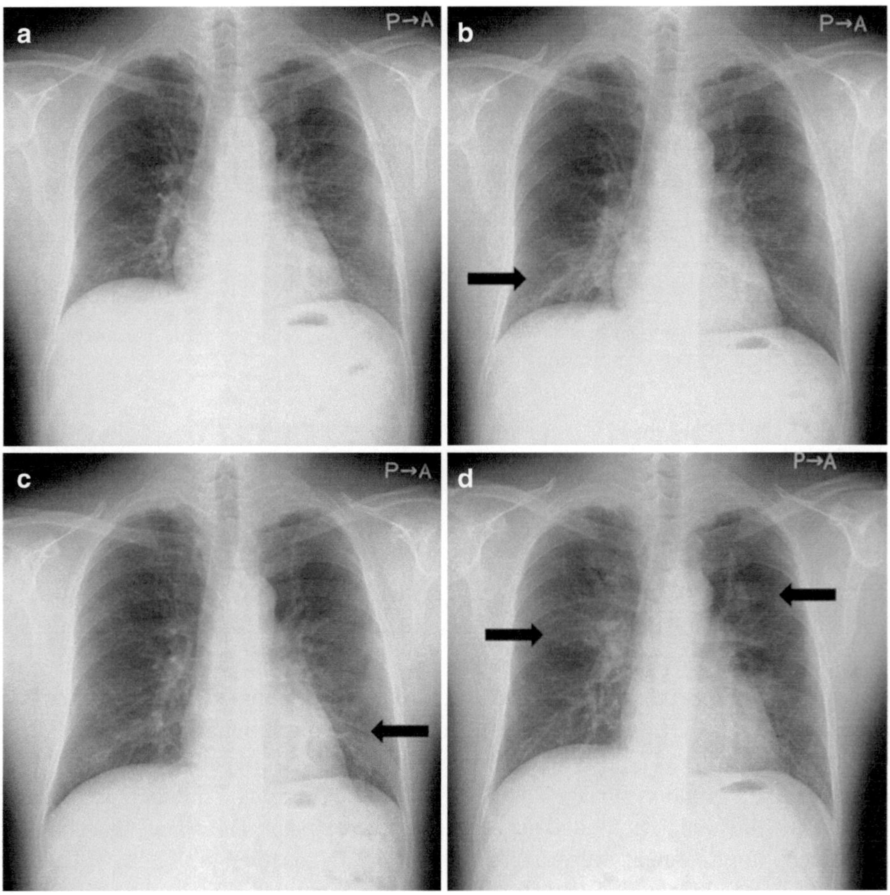

Fig. 14.6 The chest X-rays of a patient before and after the bronchial thermoplasty in our institute. (**a**) Before the treatment, (**b**) Day 2 after the first treatment (right lower lobe), (**c**) Day 2 after the second treatment (left lower lobe), (**d**) Day 2 after the third treatment (right and left upper lobe). Chest X-rays showed infiltration (arrow)

14.9 The Long-Term Efficacy and Safety of BT

Patients who were registered in the AIR, RISA, AIR2 trials were followed up for 5 years, and the efficacy and safety of BT were observed [9]. The effects with regard to reduced hospitalization, emergency visits, and severe exacerbations were maintained for 5 years. The respiratory complications and respiratory function were also well preserved.

14.10 Conclusion

BT has been used in the treatment of severe asthma; however, the mechanism of its effects and the appropriate methodology have not been fully established. It is recommended that a physician who is familiar with asthma treatment in the clinical setting and an expert in bronchoscopy choose patients appropriately. The cauterization of as much of the airway in the treatment range as possible seems to be a key to successful treatment. A multicenter study is currently underway in Japan. At present, it appears that the efficacy and the safety of BT in the real world will soon be revealed.

References

1. Chung KF, Wenzel SE, Brozek JL, et al. International ERS/ATS guidelines on definition, evaluation and treatment of severe asthma. Eur Respir J. 2014;43(2):343–73.
2. Danek CJ, Lombard CM, Dungworth DL, et al. Reduction in airway hyperresponsiveness to methacholine by the application of RF energy in dogs. J Appl Physiol (1985). 2004;97(5):1946–53.
3. Miller JD, Cox G, Vincic L, et al. A prospective feasibility study of bronchial thermoplasty in the human airway. Chest. 2005;127(6):1999–2006.
4. Cox G, Thomson NC, Rubin AS, AIR Trial Study Group, et al. Asthma control during the year after bronchial thermoplasty. N Engl J Med. 2007;356(13):1327–37.
5. Pavord ID, Cox G, Thomson NC, RISA Trial Study Group, et al. Safety and efficacy of bronchial thermoplasty in symptomatic, severe asthma. Am J Respir Crit Care Med. 2007;176(12):1185–91.
6. Castro M, Rubin AS, Laviolette M, AIR2 Trial Study Group, et al. Effectiveness and safety of bronchial thermoplasty in the treatment of severe asthma: a multicenter, randomized, double-blind, sham-controlled clinical trial. Am J Respir Crit Care Med. 2010;181(2):116–24.
7. Iikura M, Hojo M, Nagano N, et al. Bronchial thermoplasty for severe uncontrolled asthma in Japan. Allergol Int. 2018;67(2):273–5.
8. Ishii Y. Clinical usefulness of bronchial thermoplasty and its real procedure. JJSRE. 2017;39:447–52.
9. Laxmanan B, Egressy K, Murgu SD, White SR, Hogarth DK. Advances in bronchial thermoplasty. Chest. 2016;150(3):694–704.

Chapter 15
Asthma COPD Overlap (ACO)

Yasuhiro Gon, Mari Hikichi, and Shu Hashimoto

Abstract Asthma and chronic obstructive pulmonary disease (COPD) are the most common chronic airway disorders worldwide. The overlap of asthma and COPD is a problem that has been discussed for a long time, and there was previously no unified name or definition of this condition. The Global Initiative for Asthma (GINA), an international committee examining asthma, and the Global Initiative for Chronic Obstructive Lung Disease (GOLD), an international committee examining COPD, jointly proposed the concept of "Asthma/COPD Overlap Syndrome (ACOS)" (currently named "asthma/COPD overlap (ACO)." However, it is unclear how to identify ACO as a clinically useful disease entity. In this chapter, we discussed clinical features and biomarkers to differentiate asthma, COPD, and ACO in elderly patients on the basis of the definition of GINA guideline and described historical background and prevalence and treatment of ACO.

Keywords Asthma · Global Initiative for Chronic Obstructive Lung Disease (GOLD) · Asthma/COPD overlap (ACO) · Dutch hypothesis · British hypothesis

15.1 Introduction

In 1860, in his book, *Asthma*, Henry Salter proposed a concept of asthma that is similar to the one shared today [1]. However, the concept of chronic obstructive pulmonary disease (COPD) did not exist at the time when he advocated this definition of asthma. By the 1960s, debates on the differences and overlap between diseases equivalent to the current definition of COPD (e.g., chronic bronchitis,

Y. Gon (✉) · M. Hikichi · S. Hashimoto
Division of Respiratory Medicine, Department of Internal Medicine, Nihon University School of Medicine, Itabashi-ku, Tokyo, Japan
e-mail: yasuhiro.gon@nihon-u.ac.jp

A. Yokoyama (ed.), *Advances in Asthma*, Respiratory Disease Series: Diagnostic Tools and Disease Managements, https://doi.org/10.1007/978-981-13-2790-2_15

emphysema) and asthma began to develop [2, 3]. In 1961, Orie and Sluiter et al. of the Netherlands proposed a theory that asthma, chronic bronchitis, and emphysema are due to the same cause but show different expression types [4]. This is known today as the Dutch hypothesis. In contrast, in 1965, Reid et al. from the United Kingdom indicated that asthma and COPD have different causes and pathophysiology, both genetically and immunopathologically [5]. This theory is referred today as the British hypothesis and is known as a concept opposing the Dutch hypothesis [6]. Although there is no current consensus regarding the correct hypothesis, the relationship between asthma and COPD has long remained an important issue for researchers in the field.

In differential diagnosis of cases involving asthma and COPD, it is necessary to exclude COPD from the differentiated diseases for accurate diagnosis of asthma, and for accurate diagnosis of COPD, it is necessary to exclude asthma from the differentiated diseases [7, 8]. Thus, asthma and COPD can be diagnosed by mutually exclusive discrimination in the diagnostic process. However, in actual clinical practice, it is often difficult to differentiate between the two. It cannot be denied that this causes at least some confusion in diagnostic methods and selection of treatment methods in clinical practice. According to previous studies, cases of comorbid asthma and COPD have been known to have a poor prognosis [9], but large-scale clinical trials examining appropriate treatment methods for such overlapping cases have not been conducted [10].

Furthermore, in previous large clinical trials of asthma and COPD, overlapping cases tended to be unevenly excluded due to the differing exclusion criteria of each study [10]. For example, asthma patients who are smokers are always excluded from clinical trials of asthma [10]. Regarding COPD, there are clinical trials of COPD that include patients with a history of asthma as entry criteria, but there are also clinical trials that exclude such patients. Furthermore, some studies excluded patients with blood eosinophil count >600/μL, while others did not have exclusion criteria with regard to blood eosinophil count [10, 11].

Because of these reasons, there is a lack of clear evidence on the kind of treatment and management methods that are appropriate in cases of overlapping asthma and COPD. Overlap between asthma and COPD tends to increase with age [12]; with the aging of the population in recent years, this condition has increasingly become a problem that cannot be ignored. Based on this historical background in which the necessity for global recognition of the diagnosis of asthma and COPD overlap and treatment management has increased, the concept of ACO has been proposed.

15.2 The Concept of ACO

The overlap of asthma and COPD is a problem that has been discussed for a long time, and there was previously no unified name or definition of this condition. The Global Initiative for Asthma (GINA), an international committee

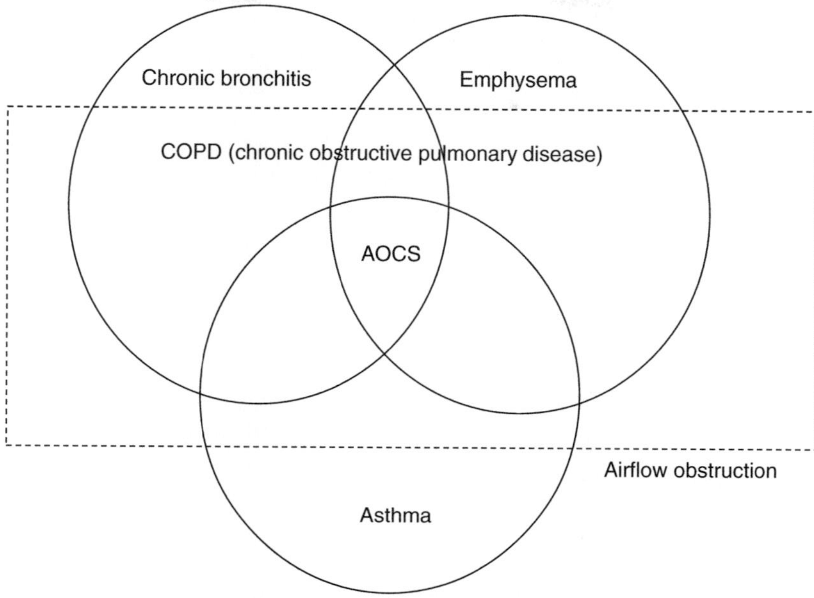

Fig. 15.1 Venn diagram showing the number of overlapping conditions in patients with asthma, emphysema, and chronic bronchitis

examining asthma, and the Global Initiative for Chronic Obstructive Lung Disease (GOLD), an international committee examining COPD, jointly proposed the concept of "Asthma/COPD Overlap Syndrome (ACOS)" in the GINA guideline in 2015 [7]. With this background, the definition of ACOS is as follows: "Asthma-COPD overlap syndrome (ACOS) is characterized by persistent airflow limitation with several features usually associated with asthma and several features usually associated with COPD [7]. Therefore, ACOS is defined as the clinical features that shares with both asthma and COPD. A specific definition for ACOS cannot be developed until more evidence is available about its clinical phenotypes and underlying mechanisms." In the subsequent revision released in 2017, "syndrome" was removed, and the name was changed to "asthma/COPD overlap (ACO)" (Fig. 15.1) [7].

15.3 Prevalence of ACO

Because there have been no clear diagnostic criteria or definitions of ACO to date, the criteria for ACO vary by study, making it difficult for a consensus to be reached. In addition, because the incidence of ACO tends to increase with age [13], the prevalence tends to be low in studies in which many younger persons are included as subjects. Furthermore, the influence of differences in countries and in study design, etc. has resulted in different results between studies.

In a survey targeting the general population, the prevalence of ACO ranged widely from 1.6% to 10.7% [14–18]. In a cohort study of 15,203 general residents aged 25 years or older as subjects, the criterion of ACO was set as a history of both asthma and COPD diagnosis in the past, and the prevalence of ACO was reported to be 2.7% [15]. In one study, the prevalence of ACO among patients with asthma was found to be 11.1–61.0% [19, 20], and in another study on the prevalence of ACO among COPD patients, the prevalence was reported to be 12.1–66.0%.

15.4 Clinical Characteristics of ACO

The symptoms of ACO are primarily cough, sputum, wheezing, shortness of breath, and dyspnoea. These symptoms are not characteristic in patients with asthma or COPD only. However, ACO is considered to cause stronger and more frequent symptoms in comparison with asthma or COPD only [21–24]. Detailed inquiries regarding triggers, patterns, persistence, progress, etc. of symptoms are diagnostic clues. Naturally, the symptoms of ACO have the characteristics of both asthma and COPD. In particular, the presence of symptoms characteristic of asthma in COPD patients provides clues for the diagnosis of ACO.

The fact that ACO patients require special management is due to the presence of the following characteristics in comparison with patients with asthma or COPD only [9, 16, 25].

1. Tendency to present with clinical symptoms
2. High frequency of exacerbation
3. Impaired QOL
4. Acceleration of lung function decline
5. High mortality rate
6. High frequency of use of mergency department visits and high medical costs

Thus, because the severity of ACO is greater than that of asthma and COPD, and the condition can be said to have a poor prognosis, proper diagnosis and management are necessary. In addition, by developing clinical studies targeting ACO, further understanding of the pathology of overlap and examination of management methods are necessary.

15.5 Diagnosis of ACO

Regarding ACO, in a document jointly published by GINA and GOLD, diagnosis of chronic respiratory tract illness was defined as Step 1, assessment of symptoms of COPD and asthma and the change in airflow obstruction as Step 2, and a stepwise approach leading to diagnosis of obstructive disorder by spirometry was proposed as Step 3 [7].

Table 15.1 Criteria for diagnosis of asthma-chronic obstructive pulmonary disease overlap syndrome

Major	Minor
1. Persistent airflow limitation (post-bronchodilator FEV_1/FVC <0.70 or LLN) in individuals 40 years of age or older; LLN is preferred 2. At least 10 pack-years of tobacco smoking *or* equivalent indoor or outdoor air pollution exposure (e.g., biomass) 3. Documented history of asthma before 40 years of age *or* BDR of >400 mL in FEV_1	1. Documented history of atopy or allergic rhinitis 2. BDR of FEV_1 ≥200 mL and 12% from baseline values on two or more visits 3. Peripheral blood eosinophil count of ≥300 cells·uL^{-1}

The committee recommends presence of all three major criteria and at least one minor criterion for asthma-chronic obstructive pulmonary disease overlap syndrome
FEV_1 forced expiratory volume in 1 s, *FVC* forced vital capacity, *BDR* bronchodilator response using 400 ug of albuterol/salbutamol (or equivalent), *LLN* lower limit of normal

On the other hand, according to the ACO diagnostic criteria proposed by Sin et al. and formulated by roundtable discussion, as shown in Table 15.1, patients with ACO fulfill the following three items: obstructive disorder revealed by spirometry, history of smoking (or exposure to air pollution) of 10 years or longer, history of asthma diagnosis at age 40 or younger, or 400 mL forced expiratory volume in 1 s (FEV1) [10]. These patients also show one of the following three findings: atopic dermatitis or allergic rhinitis, FEV1 of 200 mL or higher, or increased blood eosinophil level (>300/μL).

Both criteria and definitions have been devised to identify the characteristics of COPD and asthma and to diagnose them as ACO, but the disadvantage is that there are few objective indicators.

15.6 Biomarkers of ACO

A higher value of fractional exhaled nitric oxide (FeNO) is noted in stable patients with COPD in comparison with healthy subjects, but the value is not as high as in patients with asthma [26]. If high FeNO levels are noted in a COPD patient, the diagnostic value of ACO is considered to be high. Regarding the FeNO cutoff, in the ATS/ERS guideline reported in 2011, 25 ppb and 50 ppb are used as measures of eosinophilic airway inflammation [27]. Clinically, 25 ppb is insufficient in terms of specificity, and 50 ppb is insufficient in terms of sensitivity. Therefore, it is desirable to determine a diagnosis with reference to a certain value in between the two.

Eosinophil examination may be useful in assessing the presence of ACO in clinically diagnosed COPD patients. Previous studies have reported that sputum eosinophil count is higher in patients who receive a clinical diagnosis of COPD than in healthy subjects [28–30]. It has been reported that sputum eosinophil ratio is useful for predicting steroid reactivity, and when the sputum eosinophil ratio exceeds

3–4.5%, the efficacy of inhaled corticosteroid (ICS) or oral steroid agent is high [31, 32].

Blood eosinophil ratio and sputum eosinophil ratio show a certain correlation in case of ICS nonuse [32], and a blood eosinophil ratio of 2% is reported to correspond to sputum eosinophil ratio of 3% [33]. Elevated blood eosinophil count in COPD is highly correlated with the pathological findings of airway mucosa of asthma such as submucosal eosinophilia and basement membrane thickening, indicating that the increased elevated eosinophil count in COPD is a finding suggesting the presence of ACO [34, 35]. Regarding the relationship between high blood eosinophil count and exacerbation of condition, it has been reported that the incidence of exacerbation is high in patients with a high blood eosinophil count [36]. In addition, it was confirmed that in cases of COPD with a peripheral blood eosinophil level of 2% or more, ICS significantly inhibited exacerbation, and it is necessary to clarify how many patients fall under the criteria of ACO in the future [37].

A previous study revealed that only sputum NGAL levels could differentiate ACO from asthma and COPD [38, 39]. Sputum NGAL levels were independently correlated with the percentage of pre-bronchodilator forced expiratory volume in 1 (FEV_1) second predicted in multivariate analysis in the discovery and replication cohorts. Several studies showed that the levels of several inflammatory mediators were significantly different among the asthma only and COPD only and their overlap. Serum YKL-40 levels in the COPD and ACO group have been reported to be higher than in the asthma group [40, 41]. Sputum or serum biomarkers reflecting both airway inflammation and remodeling of the tissue show potential in differentiation between asthma, COPD, and ACO [41]. However, these studies were limited because there are currently no clear criteria for diagnosing ACO. Therefore, the utility of these molecules in sputum and serum determining levels needs further study.

15.7 ACO Treatment

There is still no consensus regarding the course of treatment of ACO that is based on adequate evidence. Therefore, at present, the appropriate treatment method of ACO is empirically selected from among the recommended treatments for asthma and COPD.

The treatment of ACO basically consists of treatment of both asthma and COPD. Since allergic airway inflammation due to comorbid asthma exists in the airway of ACO patients, ICS must be used as first-line therapy [7, 42]. The basis of asthma treatment is ICS, and the basis of COPD treatment is bronchodilator therapy with long-acting inhaled muscarinic antagonist (LAMA) or LAMA/long-acting beta-agonist (LABA), but in cases of ACO, in which both allergic inflammation and airflow obstruction are observed, it is necessary to use LABA, LAMA, or both in addition to ICS. However, in what cases is it appropriate to use ICS, how long it should be used, how to perform step down, and how to use it remain future issues to be examined.

The point to be aware of when treating ACO is to not treat with bronchodilator only, and in particular, treatment with LABA only should not be performed [43]. In ACO, in which characteristics of asthma and COPD overlap, detailed patient guidance (e.g., smoking cessation, avoidance of allergens, inhalation guidance) is indispensable, and using various questionnaires and clinical indicators used in asthma and COPD, it is necessary to understand the status of control in the patients and select therapeutic drugs accordingly. In ACO patients who experience repeated exacerbation, the causes and immunopathology of exacerbation are identified, and in severe cases, treatment using biologics such as anti-IgE antibodies or anti-IL-5 antibodies is also considered.

15.8 Conclusion: Debate Concerning the Necessity of ACO

While interest in ACO has been increasing, there are also critical opinions against regarding ACO as a single disease entity [6, 44]. The basis of the critical opinions is the view that there is a limit to defining ACO as a single pathological state or disease. Both asthma and COPD are syndromes with complicated pathologies that overlap, and regardless of how they are categorized, the indication that it is impossible to diagnose the overlapping pathologies of asthma and COPD and to accurately classify them into three disease categories is in a sense true.

However, even at the research level, accurate identification of the phenotypes or endotypes of COPD and asthma based on biomarkers is not an easy task. Furthermore, biomarkers that can be used in clinical practice are limited. In both asthma and COPD, it remains unclear as to what phenotype the disease should be classified; the concept of a phenotype/endotype-based asthma or COPD diagnosis may be a possibility in the future, but research on the subject remains incomplete. Introducing such a concept into clinical practice may be a useful suggestion for specialists, but considering the reality that the medical practitioners who treat asthma and COPD are general physicians, the possibility of confusion in clinical practice will not disappear. Therefore, the diagnosis and management of ACO as a comorbid condition rather than a phenotype is convenient and easy to understand, and it can be said that it also has clinical advantages such as broadening options for therapeutic drugs based on a disease label.

References

1. ER MF Jr. A century of asthma. Am J Respir Crit Care Med. 2004;170(3):215–21.
2. Scott JA, Mahler DA. Diagnosis of chronic obstructive pulmonary disease and differentiation from asthma. Curr Opin Pulm Med. 1995;1(2):144–9.
3. Martinez FJ. Diagnosing chronic obstructive pulmonary disease. The importance of differentiating asthma, emphysema, and chronic bronchitis. Postgrad Med. 1998;103(4):112–7. 121–2, 125.

4. Orie NGM, Sluiter HJ, de Vries K, Tammeling GJ, Witkop J. The host factor in bronchitis. In: Orie NGM, Sluiter HJ, editors. Bronchitis. Assen: Royal van. Gorcum; 1961. p. 43–59.
5. Reid L. The role of chronic bronchitis in the production of "chronic obstructive pulmonary emphysema". J Am Med Womens Assoc. 1965;20:633–8.
6. Soler X, Ramsdell JW. Are asthma and COPD a continuum of the same disease? J Allergy Clin Immunol Pract. 2015;3(4):489–95.
7. Global initiative for asthma. Global strategy for asthma management and prevention. 2017. http://ginasthma.org/2017-gina-report-global-strategy-for-asthma-management-and-prevention/.
8. Global strategy for the diagnosis, Management and prevention of chronic obstructive pulmonary disease (GOLD). 2017.
9. Silva GE, Sherrill DL, Guerra S, Barbee RA. Asthma as a risk factor for COPD in a longitudinal study. Chest. 2004;126(1):59–65.
10. Sin DD, Miravitlles M, Mannino DM, Soriano JB, Price D, Celli BR, Leung JM, Nakano Y, Park HY, Wark PA, Wechsler ME. What is asthma-COPD overlap syndrome? Towards a consensus definition from a round table discussion. Eur Respir J. 2016;48(3):664–73.
11. Wedzicha JA, Banerji D, Chapman KR, Vestbo J, Roche N, Ayers RT, Thach C, Fogel R, Patalano F, Vogelmeier CF, FLAME Investigators. Indacaterol-Glycopyrronium versus Salmeterol-fluticasone for COPD. N Engl J Med. 2016;374(23):2222–34.
12. Gibson PG, McDonald VM. Asthma-COPD overlap 2015: now we are six. Thorax. 2015;70(7):683–91.
13. Soriano JB, Davis KJ, Coleman B, et al. The proportional Venn diagram of obstructive lung disease: two approximations from the United States and the United Kingdom. Chest. 2003;124:474–81.
14. de Marco R, Marcon A, Rossi A, et al. Asthma, COPD and overlap syndrome: a longitudinal study in young European adults. Eur Respir J. 2015;46:671–9.
15. Diaz-Guzman E, Khosravi M, Mannino DM. Asthma, chronic obstructive pulmonary disease, and mortality in the U.S. population. COPD. 2011;8:400–7.
16. Menezes AM, Montes de Oca M, Pérez-Padilla R, et al. Increased risk of exacerbation and hospitalization in subjects with an overlap phenotype: COPD-asthma. Chest. 2014;145:297–304.
17. de Marco R, Pesce G, Marcon A, et al. The coexistence of asthma and chronic obstructive pulmonary disease (COPD): prevalence and risk factors in young, middle-aged and elderly people from the general population. PLoS One. 2013;8:e62985.
18. Shirtcliffe P, Marsh S, Travers J, et al. Childhood asthma and GOLD-defined chronic obstructive pulmonary disease. Intern Med J. 2012;42(1):83–8.
19. Wurst KE, Kelly-Reif K, Bushnell GA, et al. Understanding asthma-chronic obstructive pulmonary disease overlap syndrome. Respir Med. 2016;110:1–11.
20. Tamada T, Sugiura H, Takahashi T, et al. Biomarker-based detection of asthma-COPD overlap syndrome in COPD populations. Int J Chron Obstruct Pulmon Dis. 2015;10:2169–76.
21. Alshabanat A, Zafari Z, Albanyan O, et al. Asthma and COPD overlap syndrome (ACOS): a systematic review and meta analysis. PLoS One. 2015;10:e0136065.
22. Pascoe S, Locantore N, Dransfield MT, et al. Blood eosinophil counts, exacerbations, and response to the addition of inhaled fluticasone furoate to vilanterol in patients with chronic obstructive pulmonary disease: a secondary analysis of data from two parallel randomised controlled trials. Lancet Respir Med. 2015;3:435–42.
23. Cosio BG, Soriano JB, López-Campos JL, et al. Defining the asthma-COPD overlap syndrome in a COPD cohort. Chest. 2016;149:45–52.
24. Hardin M, Cho M, McDonald ML, et al. The clinical and genetic features of COPD-asthma overlap syndrome. Eur Respir J. 2014;44:341–50.
25. Miravitlles M, Soriano JB, Ancochea J, et al. Characterisation of the overlap COPD-asthma phenotype. Focus on physical activity and health status. Respir Med. 2013;107:1053–60.
26. Ichinose M, Sugiura H, Yamagata S, et al. Increase in reactive nitrogen species production in chronic obstructive pulmonary disease airways. Am J Respir Crit Care Med. 2000;162:701–6.

27. Dweik RA, Boggs PB, Erzurum SC, et al. An official ATS clinical practice guideline:interpretation of exhaled nitric oxide levels (FENO) for clinical applications. Am J Respir Crit Care Med. 2011;184:602–15.
28. Rutgers SR, Timens W, Kaufmann HF, et al. Comparison of induced sputum with bronchial wash, bronchoalveolar lavage and bronchial biopsies in COPD. Eur Respir J. 2000;15:109–15.
29. Eltboli O, Bafadhel M, Hollins F, et al. COPD exacerbation severity and frequency is associated with impaired macrophage efferocytosis of eosinophils. BMC Pulm Med. 2014;14:112.
30. Pizzichini E, Pizzichini MM, Gibson P, et al. Sputum eosinophilia predicts benefit from prednisone in smokers with chronic obstructive bronchitis. Am J Respir Crit Care Med. 1998;158:1511–7.
31. Brightling CE, Monteiro W, Ward R, et al. Sputum eosinophilia and short-term response to prednisolone in chronic obstructive pulmonary disease:a randomised controlled trial. Lancet. 2000;356:1480–5.
32. Brightling CE, McKenna S, Hargadon B, et al. Sputum eosinophilia and the short term response to inhaled mometasone in chronic obstructive pulmonary disease. Thorax. 2005;60:193–8.
33. Bafadhel M, McKenna S, Terry S, et al. Acute exacerbations of chronic obstructive pulmonary disease:identification of biologic clusters and their biomarkers. Am J Respir Crit Care Med. 2011;184:662–71.
34. Kolsum U, Damera G, Pham TH, Southworth T, Mason S, Karur P, Newbold P, Singh D. Pulmonary inflammation in patients with chronic obstructive pulmonary disease with higher blood eosinophil counts. J Allergy Clin Immunol. 2017;140(4):1181–1184.e7.
35. Eltboli O, Mistry V, Barker B, et al. Relationship between blood and bronchial submucosal eosinophilia and reticular basement membrane thickening in chronic obstructive pulmonary disease. Respirology. 2015;20:667–70.
36. Vedel-Krogh S, Nielsen SF, Lange P, et al. Blood eosinophils and exacerbations in chronic obstructive pulmonary disease. The copenhagen general population study. Am J Respir Crit Care Med. 2016;193:965–74.
37. Singh D, Kolsum U, Brightling CE, et al. Eosinophilic inflammation in COPD:prevalence and clinical characteristics. Eur Respir J. 2014;44:1697–700.
38. Iwamoto H, Gao J, Koskela J, Kinnula V, Kobayashi H, Laitinen T, Mazur W. Differences in plasma and sputum biomarkers between COPD and COPD-asthma overlap. Eur Respir J. 2014;43(2):421–9.
39. Gao J, Iwamoto H, Koskela J, Alenius H, Hattori N, Kohno N, Laitinen T, Mazur W, Pulkkinen V. Characterization of sputum biomarkers for asthma-COPD overlap syndrome. Int J Chron Obstruct Pulmon Dis. 2016;30(11):2457–65.
40. James AJ, Reinius LE, Verhoek M, Gomes A, Kupczyk M, Hammar U, Ono J, Ohta S, Izuhara K, Bel E, Kere J, Söderhäll C, Dahlén B, Boot RG, Dahlén SE, BIOAIR (Longitudinal Assessment of Clinical Course and Biomarkers in Severe Chronic Airway Disease) Consortium. Increased YKL-40 and Chitotriosidase in asthma and chronic obstructive pulmonary disease. Am J Respir Crit Care Med. 2016;193(2):131–42.
41. Gon Y, Maruoka S, Ito R, Mizumura K, Kozu Y, Hiranuma H, Hattori T, Takahashi M, Hikichi M, Hashimoto S. Utility of serum YKL-40 levels for identification of patients with asthma and COPD. Allergol Int. 2017;66(4):624–6.
42. Ichinose M. Asthma prevention and management guideline 2015. Arerugi. 2017;66(2):77–81.
43. Salpeter SR, Buckley NS, Ormiston TM, et al. Meta-analysis: effect of long-acting beta-agonists on severe asthma exacerbations and asthma-related deaths. Ann Intern Med. 2006;144:904–12.
44. Bateman ED, Reddel HK, van Zyl-Smit RN, Agusti A. The asthma-COPD overlap syndrome: towards a revised taxonomy of chronic airways diseases? Lancet Respir Med. 2015;3(9):719–28.

Chapter 16
Future Treatment and Other New Biologics for Asthma

Hiroshi Ohnishi and Akihito Yokoyama

Abstract Various cytokines and their receptors implicated in asthma pathophysiology are new targets for future treatments for severe asthma. There are several asthma endotypes that are characterized by the presence of (1) immunoglobulin E (IgE)-mediated inflammation, (2) type 2 inflammation (T2)-high, and (3) T2-low. Endotype-based approaches are new therapeutic strategies for severe asthma. In some countries, monoclonal antibodies (mAbs) that block IgE or interleukin (IL)-5 signaling are being used to treat severe allergic asthma and severe eosinophilic asthma, respectively. Neutralizing mAbs that target the IL-4/IL-13 signaling pathway and thymic stromal lymphopoietin (TSLP) were investigated in several clinical trials involving patients with severe asthma. Drugs generated from these mAbs, such as dupilumab and tezepelumab, may be promising treatments for severe asthma patients. An antagonist of the chemoattractant receptor-homologous molecule on Th2 cells (CRTh2) is another promising drug for the treatment of asthma. Macrolides are also effective for reducing asthma exacerbation in patients with severe asthma. Together, these therapies hold promise for more effective management of asthma.

Keywords Biologic · Chemoattractant receptor-homologous molecule on Th2 cells (CRTh2) · IL-4 · IL-5 · IL-13 · Macrolide · Severe asthma · Thymic stromal lymphopoietin (TSLP)

H. Ohnishi (✉) · A. Yokoyama
Department of Hematology and Respiratory Medicine, Kochi Medical School, Kochi University, Nankoku, Kochi, Japan
e-mail: honi@kochi-u.ac.jp

A. Yokoyama (ed.), *Advances in Asthma*, Respiratory Disease Series: Diagnostic Tools and Disease Managements, https://doi.org/10.1007/978-981-13-2790-2_16

Abbreviations

ACQ	Asthma control questionnaire
ADCC	Antibody-dependent cell cytotoxicity
AQLQ	Asthma quality of life questionnaire
AZM	Azithromycin
CRTh2	Chemoattractant receptor-homologous molecule on Th2 cells
EGPA	Eosinophilic granulomatosis with polyangiitis
FDA	Food and Drug Administration
FeNO	Fraction of exhaled nitric oxide
FEV1	Forced expiratory volume in 1 second
ICS	Inhaled corticosteroids
IgE	Immunoglobulin E
IL	Interleukin
ILC2	Group 2 innate lymphoid cells
LABA	Long-acting β2 agonist
LAMA	Long-acting muscarinic antagonist
mAb	Monoclonal antibody
OCS	Oral corticosteroids
QOL	Quality of life
Th2	Type 2 helper T
TSLP	Thymic stromal lymphopoietin

16.1 Introduction

Various cytokines such as type 2 helper T (Th2) cytokines and their receptors, thymic stromal lymphopoietin (TSLP), and chemoattractant receptor-homologous molecule on Th2 cells (CRTh2) play important roles in asthma pathophysiology and are new therapeutic targets for severe asthma [1]. Recent treatment strategies for severe asthma are based on stratification of asthma endotypes: (1) immunoglobulin E (IgE)-mediated inflammation, (2) type 2 inflammation (T2)-high, and (3) T2-low. Omalizumab, an anti-IgE monoclonal antibody (mAb), is the first biologic used to treat severe allergic asthma that reduces asthma exacerbation and improves lung function and health-related quality of life (QOL) [2]. T2-high asthma is driven by Th2 cytokines such as interleukin (IL)-4, IL-5, and IL-13 and is characterized by eosinophilia in the blood and/or sputum, increased fraction of exhaled nitric oxide (FeNO), and/or high serum periostin concentration [3]. Blockage of IL-4, IL-5, IL-13, and TSLP signaling by mAbs is a new approach for treatment of T2-high asthma. The effects of blocking mAbs for cytokines and their receptors that are used to treat T2-high severe asthma are summarized in Table 16.1. In this chapter, we review promising future drugs for severe asthma.

Table 16.1 Summary of effects of major biologics for T2-high severe asthma

Type of biologics	Drug name	Target	Biomarkers	Effects of biologics							Reference #
				Asthma exacerbation	FEV1	QOL	FeNO	Blood eosinophils	Serum IgE level	Other effects	
Anti-IgE mAb	Omalizumab	Allergic asthma	FeNO high, serum periostin-high, blood eosinophils ≥300/μL	Reduced	Small increased	Improved	Decreased	Decreased	Total IgE was increased, but free IgE was decreased	Inhibition of airway remodeling	[2]
Anti-IL-5 mAb	Mepolizumab	Severe eosinophilic asthma	Blood eosinophils ≥150/μL	Reduced	Increased	Improved	Not decreased in a small study	Decreased	No change	Oral corticosteroid sparing in severe eosinophilic asthma and EGPA	[4–9]
	Reslizumab	Severe eosinophilic asthma	Blood eosinophils ≥400/μL	Reduced	Increased	Improved	No data	Decreased	No data		[10]
Anti-IL-5Rα mAb	Benralizumab	Severe eosinophilic asthma	Blood eosinophils ≥300/μL	Reduced	Increased	Improved	Not decreased in a small study	Decreased	No data	Oral corticosteroid sparing	[11–15]
Anti-IL-13 mAb	Lebrikizumab	Uncontrolled asthma	Serum periostin-high, FeNO high	Not consistent data	Increased	Not consistent data	Decreased	Increased	Decreased in another study		[16, 17]
	Tralokinumab	Severe uncontrolled asthma	Serum periostin-high, serum DPP4 high, FeNO high	Negative data	Increased in some group	Not improved	No data	Increased	No data		[18]

(continued)

Table 16.1 (continued)

Type of biologics	Drug name	Target	Biomarkers	Effects of biologics							Reference #
				Asthma exacerbation	FEV1	QOL	FeNO	Blood eosinophils	Serum IgE level	Other effects	
Anti-IL-4Rα mAb	Dupilumab	Severe uncontrolled asthma	Blood eosinophils ≥300/μL	Reduced	Increased	Improved	Decreased	Increased	Decreased		[19]
Anti-TSLP mAb	Tezepelumab	Uncontrolled asthma	Unknown	Reduced	Increased	Improved in high dose	Decreased	Decreased	Decreased	Inhibition of antigen-induced airway hyperresponsiveness	[20, 21]

DPP4 Dipeptidyl peptidase-4, *EGPA* eosinophilic granulomatosis with polyangiitis, *FeNO* fraction of exhaled nitric oxide, *FEV1* forced expiratory volume in one second, *IgE* immunoglobulin E, *IL* interleukin, *QOL* quality of life, *TSLP* thymic stromal lymphopoietin

16.2 IL-5 Targeting Therapy

IL-5 is produced by Th2 cells, group 2 innate lymphoid cells (ILC2), mast cells, $CD34^+$ bone marrow stem cells, invariant natural killer T cells, and eosinophils. IL-5 binding to IL-5 receptor α (IL-5Rα) induces differentiation, maturation, migration, and degranulation of eosinophils [22]. Increased eosinophilic airway inflammation is associated with more frequent asthma exacerbation events, which can be reduced by anti-IL-5 mAb therapy. Mepolizumab and reslizumab are anti-IL-5 mAbs that decrease the number of circulating eosinophils but may not eliminate these cells in the airway. Benralizumab is an afucosylated anti-IL-5Rα mAb that augments interactions with Fcγ receptors expressed on natural killer cells, macrophages, and neutrophils and therefore induces antibody-dependent cell cytotoxicity (ADCC) and more effectively depletes eosinophils in the airway (Fig. 16.1).

16.2.1 Mepolizumab

Mepolizumab is a humanized monoclonal antibody (mAb) of the IgG1 kappa subclass that can be administered subcutaneously and has a good safety profile. This mAb significantly reduced asthma exacerbations in the DREAM and MENSA studies and showed oral corticosteroid (OCS)-sparing effect in the SIRIUS study [4–6].

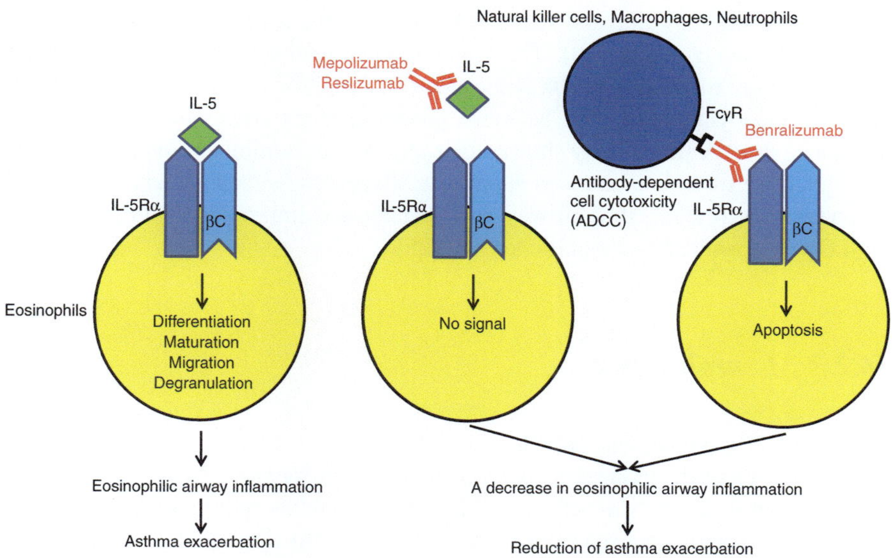

Fig. 16.1 IL-5 signaling and biologics. IL-5 binds to the IL-5 receptor α (IL-5Rα) and induces eosinophil activation, which is associated with asthma exacerbation. Mepolizumab or reslizumab block IL-5 binding, whereas benralizumab induces eosinophil apoptosis through antibody-dependent cell cytotoxicity (ADCC)

In the MUSCA study involving patients with severe eosinophilic asthma, mepolizumab treatment improved asthma symptoms, QOL, and forced expiratory volume in 1 second (FEV1) [7]. Clinically significant reductions in asthma exacerbations were noted at baseline blood eosinophil counts of ≥150 cells/μL, and this cutoff value can serve as a biomarker to select patients who may respond to mepolizumab [8]. Importantly, the effect of mepolizumab in reducing asthma exacerbations is not dependent on prior use of omalizumab [23]. Neutralization of IL-5 binding by mepolizumab reduced but did not completely eradicate asthma exacerbations. Mepolizumab reduced the number of airway eosinophils, but the remaining cells retained function [24]. The use of mepolizumab as an add-on therapy for severe asthma patients aged 12 years or older has been approved in the United States, Europe, and Japan. Mepolizumab reduced OCS use and improved the proportion and accrued time of remission in patients with eosinophilic granulomatosis with polyangiitis (EGPA) [9]. The US Food and Drug Administration (FDA) has since expanded use of mepolizumab for treatment of adult EGPA patients.

16.2.2 Reslizumab

In phase 3 trials, reslizumab, a humanized anti-IL-5 mAb of the IgG4 kappa subclass administered intravenously, significantly reduced asthma exacerbations and improved FEV1 while also improving scores on the Asthma Control Questionnaire (ACQ) and Asthma Quality of Life Questionnaire (AQLQ) in patients with inadequately controlled asthma and blood eosinophil counts ≥400 cells/μL, which predicts airway eosinophilia [10]. The US FDA approved reslizumab for use as an add-on therapy for adult patients with severe eosinophilic asthma. Reslizumab can produce anaphylaxis but may be more potent in terms of improved FEV1 and asthma control. A small study showed that intravenous administration of a weight-adjusted dose of reslizumab was superior to fixed-dose subcutaneous delivery of mepolizumab in attenuating airway eosinophilia and improving ACQ in patients with OCS-dependent eosinophilic asthma [25].

16.2.3 Benralizumab

Benralizumab, a humanized anti-IL-5Rα mAb of the IgG1 kappa subclass administered subcutaneously, induces eosinophil and basophil apoptosis by ADCC to eliminate eosinophils not only in peripheral blood but also in the sputum and airways and in turn significantly reduces asthma exacerbations [26] (Fig. 16.1). The ZONDA study showed an OCS-sparing effect of benralizumab and reduced asthma exacerbation in patients with severe asthma [11]. The SIROCCO and CALIMA study showed greater improvements associated with benralizumab used to treat acute exacerbations, as well as improved FEV1, ACQ, and AQLQ in severe uncontrolled asthma patients with high blood eosinophil levels of ≥300 cells/μL and a history of more frequent exacerbations [12–14]. Benralizumab reduced asthma exacerbations, improved symptoms, increased FEV1, and was well-tolerated in a study involving Japanese patients with severe, uncontrolled eosinophilic asthma [15]. However, the phase 3 BISE study did not show a clinically important difference of ≥10% in FEV1 or differences in other parameters for patients with mild-to-moderate persistent asthma treated with benralizumab [27]. As such, benralizumab has been approved by the US FDA as an add-on treatment for severe eosinophilic asthma.

16.3 IL-4/IL-13 Targeting Therapy

IL-4 and IL-13 are secreted mainly from $CD4^+$ Th2 cells and ILC2 and play a central role in pathophysiology of T2-high asthma through promotion of IgE production via an IgE class switch in plasma cells, enhancement of airway smooth muscle contractility, chemokine induction-dependent airway recruitment of eosinophils, airway hyperresponsiveness, and airway remodeling such as goblet cell hyperplasia, myofibroblast transformation, collagen deposition, and proliferation of airway smooth muscle cells.

IL-4 exerts strong inflammatory responses not only through the type I receptor composed of a IL-4Rα and common gamma chain (γC) heterodimer expressed on immune/inflammatory cells but also via airway structural responses by binding to type II receptors (IL-4Rα and IL-13Rα1 heterodimer) widely expressed at low levels on most cell types, including structural resident airway cells (Fig. 16.2). On the other hand, IL-13 exerts mainly airway structural responses by binding to type II receptors. IL-13 also binds to IL-13Rα2, which does not participate in signaling but instead acts as a decoy receptor [28, 29]. Inhibition of IL-4Rα binding blocks both IL-4 and IL-13 function, including immune responses and airway structural changes. On the other hand, inhibition of IL-13 binding to receptors reduces airway structural changes but affects immune responses to a lesser degree. These differences may explain why the anti-IL-4Rα mAb dupilumab (see below) has multiple positive effects for treatment of severe asthma but the anti-IL-13 mAbs lebrikizumab or tralokinumab (see below) do not. Both periostin and FeNO are expressed downstream of IL-4/IL-13 signaling and could be potential biomarkers for selecting patients with high IL-4/IL-13 status. In contrast, eosinophil count is not a direct predictor of anti-IL-13 or anti-IL-4Rα mAb success, because these mAbs do not block IL-5 action. Moreover, blocking mAbs that target IL-4/IL-13 signaling may inhibit chemokine-induced airway recruitment of eosinophils and therefore cause a transient rise of blood eosinophil counts in asthma patients. As such, caution is needed when treating patients who have high blood eosinophil counts after receiving these mAbs. Biomarkers that can predict dupilumab response are not known, but FeNO produced by inducible nitric oxide synthase in the bronchial epithelium or serum periostin levels may serve as a biomarker. Individual IL-4- and IL-13-targeting mAbs are discussed below.

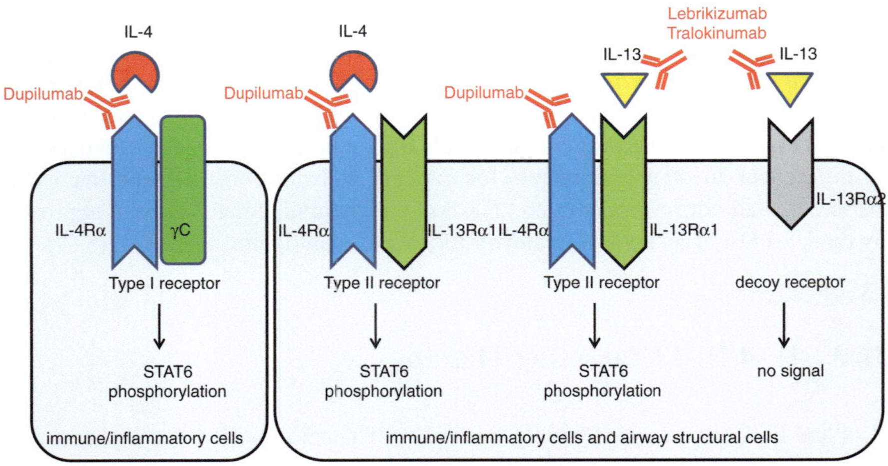

Fig. 16.2 IL-4 and IL-13 signaling pathway and biologics. IL-4 binds to both type I and type II receptors (IL-4Rα and common gamma chain (γC) heterodimer and IL-4Rα and IL-13Rα1 heterodimer, respectively). The γC subunit is primarily expressed on immune/inflammatory cells such as B lymphocytes, dendritic cells, monocytes/macrophages, eosinophils, and basophils. IL-4Rα and IL-13Rα1 are expressed at low levels on most cells, including immune cells and structural airway cells such as endothelial cells, bronchial epithelial cells, fibroblasts, and airway smooth muscle cells. IL-4 binds IL-4Rα with high affinity, but IL-13 binds IL-13Rα1 with lower affinity than that of IL-4/IL-4Rα, resulting in competition for type II receptor binding. IL-13 binds to IL-13Rα1 with low affinity or to the decoy receptor IL-13Rα2. Dupilumab blocks both IL-4 and IL-13 signaling. Lebrikizumab and tralokinumab block IL-13 signaling

16.3.1 Lebrikizumab

In a phase 2 study, lebrikizumab, a humanized anti-IL-13 mAb of the IgG4 subclass, reduced asthma exacerbation and improved FEV1 in patients with uncontrolled asthma, particularly in patients with high concentrations of the T2 biomarker periostin or a high number of blood eosinophils [16]. However, lebrikizumab did not consistently and significantly reduce asthma exacerbations in uncontrolled asthma patients with high levels of T2-high biomarkers in LAVOLTA I and LAVOLTA II phase 3 trials [17]. This mAb is no longer under investigation for treatment of asthma patients.

16.3.2 Tralokinumab

Tralokinumab, a human anti-IL-13 neutralizing mAb of the IgG4 subclass, failed to show clinical benefits such as reduced asthma exacerbations in patients with severe uncontrolled asthma [18]. Moreover, phase 3 STROTOS1, STRATOS2, and TROPOS trials showed that tralokinumab did not achieve a significant reduction in asthma exacerbation or OCS use in patients with severe uncontrolled asthma (announcement from the developer; data not yet published as of Dec 2017).

16.3.3 Anti-IL-4Rα mAb Dupilumab

Dupilumab, a human anti-IL-4Rα mAb of the IgG4 subclass, inhibits both IL-4 and IL-13 signaling, which are key drivers of T2 inflammation. Dupilumab increased FEV1, reduced asthma exacerbations, and improved ACQ and AQLQ in patients with persistent uncontrolled asthma who received medium-to-high dose inhaled corticosteroids (ICS) plus a long-acting β2 agonist (LABA), irrespective of baseline blood eosinophil count [19]. Dupilumab is currently available for treatment of moderate-to-severe atopic dermatitis, but not for asthma. However, recent data suggest that dupilumab is a promising biologic for treatment of severe uncontrolled asthma irrespective of baseline blood eosinophil count.

16.4 Anti-TSLP mAb Tezepelumab

TSLP is a bronchial epithelial cell-derived cytokine released in response to environmental and inflammatory stimuli and initiates T2 inflammation. Tezepelumab, a human anti-TSLP mAb of the IgG2 subclass, reduced airway hyperresponsiveness and airway inflammation after allergen challenge in patients with mild allergic asthma [20]. Moreover, tezepelumab reduced asthma exacerbations irrespective of baseline blood eosinophil counts, FeNO, or serum IgE levels in asthma patients treated with medium-to high doses of ICS plus LABA. Tezepelumab also increased FEV1 and reduced FeNO levels, serum IgE levels, and blood eosinophil counts [21]. These changes in biomarkers also support that TSLP acts as an upstream cytokine that influences cytokines in the Th2 pathway including IL-4, IL-5, and IL-13. Targeting TSLP is thus a promising treatment for various asthmas that are triggered not by only allergens but also viruses, tobacco smoke, and diesel exhaust.

16.5 CRTh2 Targeting Therapy

Prostaglandin D2 binds to CRTh2, also known as DP2 receptor, expressed on Th2 cells, ILC2, eosinophils, and basophils to induce chemotaxis of these inflammatory cells to the airway during allergic inflammation. Fevipiprant, a CRTh2 antagonist, reduced eosinophilic airway inflammation in patients with persistent moderate-to-severe asthma and sputum eosinophilia, despite ICS treatment, and had a favorable safety profile [30]. Fevipiprant improved FEV1 in allergic asthma that was uncontrolled on low-dose ICS treatment, but further investigations to show clinical benefits of the use of fevipiprant for asthma patients are warranted [31].

16.6 Macrolides

In the AMAZE study, add-on therapy with the macrolide 500 mg azithromycin (AZM) three times per week for 48 weeks significantly reduced asthma exacerbations regardless of eosinophilic or non-eosinophilic status and improved AQLQ and ACQ in adult patients with persistent uncontrolled asthma on maintenance treatment with medium-to-high dose ICS plus LABA or a long-acting muscarinic antagonist (LAMA). The major side effect of AZM was diarrhea. Although there was a nonsignificant increase in the numbers of AZM-resistant bacteria in sputum samples, use of AZM should nonetheless be restricted to asthma patients with frequent exacerbations and avoided for patients with prolonged QT interval [32].

16.7 Summary and Conclusions

Treatment of severe asthma begins with confirmation of diagnosis followed by assessment of adherence and inhaler device handling, avoidance of allergens, smoking cessation, treating coexisting comorbidities, and add-on therapy with LABA, LAMA, leukotriene receptor antagonist, and/or theophylline, if these compounds are not already in use (Fig. 16.3). Targeting IL-5 signaling and eosinophils by the mAbs mepolizumab, reslizumab, or benralizumab is effective for reducing asthma exacerbation in patients with severe eosinophilic asthma. Severe eosinophilic asthma complicated with eosinophilic chronic eosinophilic rhinosinusitis, eosinophilic otitis media, EGPA, or chronic eosinophilic pneumonia are possible therapeutic targets of these mAbs. Blockage of IL-4Rα signaling by dupilumab is a promising add-on treatment for T2-high severe asthma irrespective of blood eosinophilia. Targeting TSLP with tezepelumab may be effective for a wide variety of uncontrolled asthma. CRTh2 antagonists are also promising as a new oral medication for asthma. Macrolides are effective for reducing asthma exacerbation irrespective of eosinophilic or non-eosinophilic asthma. Further clinical studies are needed to identify biomarkers that can be used to predict response to the variety of available asthma treatments.

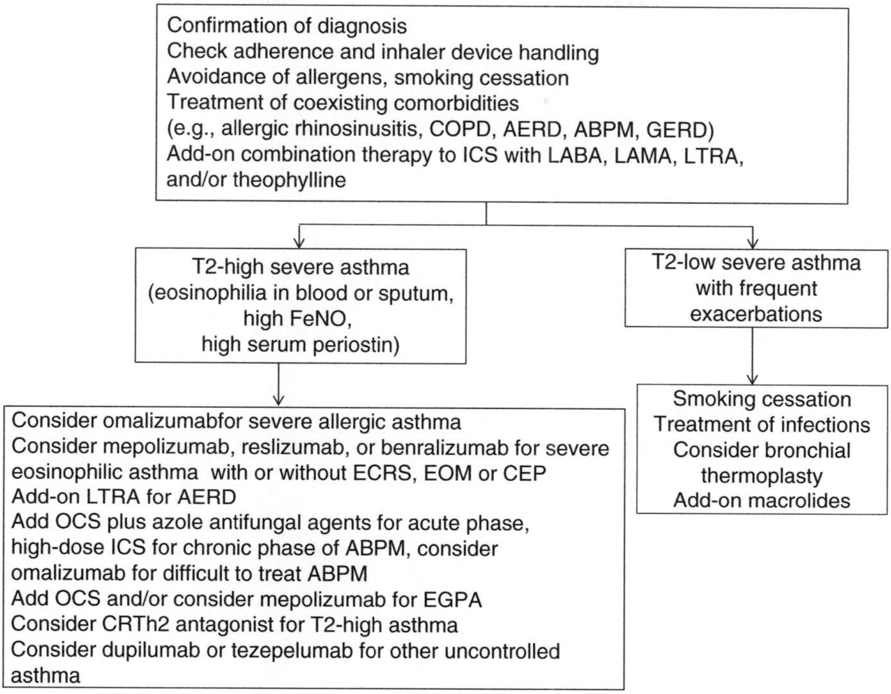

Fig. 16.3 Possible strategy for future treatment of severe asthma by biologics and other drugs. *ABPM* allergic bronchopulmonary mycosis, *AERD* aspirin-exacerbated respiratory disease, *COPD* chronic obstructive pulmonary disease, *CEP* chronic eosinophilic pneumonia, *ECRS* eosinophilic chronic rhinosinusitis, *EGPA* eosinophilic granulomatosis with polyangiitis, *EOM* eosinophilic otitis media, *FeNO* fraction of exhaled nitric oxide, *GERD* gastroesophageal reflux disease, *ICS* inhaled corticosteroid, *LABA* long-acting β2 agonist, *LAMA* long-acting muscarinic antagonist, *LTRA* leukotriene receptor antagonist, *OCS* oral corticosteroid, *T2* Type 2 inflammation

References

1. Chung KF. Asthma phenotyping: a necessity for improved therapeutic precision and new targeted therapies. J Intern Med. 2016;279:192–204.
2. Normansell R, Walker S, Milan SJ, et al. Omalizumab for asthma in adults and children. Cochrane Database Syst Rev. 2014;1:CD003559.
3. Swedin L, Saarne T, Rehnberg M, et al. Patient stratification and the unmet need in asthma. Pharmacol Ther. 2017;169:13–34.
4. Pavord ID, Korn S, Howarth P, et al. Mepolizumab for severe eosinophilic asthma (DREAM): a multicentre, double-blind, placebo-controlled trial. Lancet. 2012;380:651–9.
5. Ortega HG, Liu MC, Pavord ID, et al. Mepolizumab treatment in patients with severe eosinophilic asthma. N Engl J Med. 2014;371:1198–207.

6. Bel EH, Wenzel SE, Thompson PJ, et al. Oral glucocorticoid-sparing effect of mepolizumab in eosinophilic asthma. N Engl J Med. 2014;371:1189–97.
7. Chupp GL, Bradford ES, Albers FC, et al. Efficacy of mepolizumab add-on therapy on health-related quality of life and markers of asthma control in severe eosinophilic asthma (MUSCA): a randomised, double-blind, placebo-controlled, parallel-group, multicentre, phase 3b trial. Lancet Respir Med. 2017;5:390–400.
8. Ortega HG, Yancey SW, Mayer B, et al. Severe eosinophilic asthma treated with mepolizumab stratified by baseline eosinophil thresholds: a secondary analysis of the DREAM and MENSA studies. Lancet Respir Med. 2016;4:549–56.
9. Wechsler ME, Akuthota P, Jayne D, et al. Mepolizumab or placebo for eosinophilic granulomatosis with polyangiitis. N Engl J Med. 2017;376:1921–32.
10. Castro M, Zangrilli J, Wechsler ME, et al. Reslizumab for inadequately controlled asthma with elevated blood eosinophil counts: results from two multicentre, parallel, double-blind, randomised, placebo-controlled, phase 3 trials. Lancet Respir Med. 2015;3:355–66.
11. Nair P, Wenzel S, Rabe KF, et al. Oral glucocorticoid-sparing effect of benralizumab in severe asthma. N Engl J Med. 2017;376:2448–58.
12. FitzGerald JM, Bleecker ER, Nair P, et al. Benralizumab, an anti-interleukin-5 receptor α monoclonal antibody, as add-on treatment for patients with severe, uncontrolled, eosinophilic asthma (CALIMA): a randomised, double-blind, placebo-controlled phase 3 trial. Lancet. 2016;388:2128–41.
13. Bleecker ER, FitzGerald JM, Chanez P, et al. Efficacy and safety of benralizumab for patients with severe asthma uncontrolled with high-dosage inhaled corticosteroids and long-acting β2-agonists (SIROCCO): a randomised, multicentre, placebo-controlled phase 3 trial. Lancet. 2016;388:2115–27.
14. FitzGerald JM, Bleecker ER, Menzies-Gow A, et al. Predictors of enhanced response with benralizumab for patients with severe asthma: pooled analysis of the SIROCCO and CALIMA studies. Lancet Respir Med. 2018;6(1):51–64.
15. Ohta K, Adachi M, Tohda Y, et al. Efficacy and safety of benralizumab in Japanese patients with severe, uncontrolled eosinophilic asthma. Allergol Int. 2018;67(2):266–72.
16. Hanania NA, Noonan M, Corren J, et al. Lebrikizumab in moderate-to-severe asthma: pooled data from two randomised placebo-controlled studies. Thorax. 2015;70:748–56.
17. Hanania NA, Korenblat P, Chapman KR, et al. Efficacy and safety of lebrikizumab in patients with uncontrolled asthma (LAVOLTA I and LAVOLTA II): replicate, phase 3, randomised, double-blind, placebo-controlled trials. Lancet Respir Med. 2016;4:781–96.
18. Brightling CE, Chanez P, Leigh R, et al. Efficacy and safety of tralokinumab in patients with severe uncontrolled asthma: a randomised, double-blind, placebo-controlled, phase 2b trial. Lancet Respir Med. 2015;3:692–701.
19. Wenzel S, Castro M, Corren J, et al. Dupilumab efficacy and safety in adults with uncontrolled persistent asthma despite use of medium-to-high-dose inhaled corticosteroids plus a long-acting β2 agonist: a randomised double-blind placebo-controlled pivotal phase 2b dose-ranging trial. Lancet. 2016;388:31–44.
20. Gauvreau GM, O'Byrne PM, Boulet LP, et al. Effects of an anti-TSLP antibody on allergen-induced asthmatic responses. N Engl J Med. 2014;370:2102–10.
21. Corren J, Parnes JR, Wang L, et al. Tezepelumab in adults with uncontrolled asthma. N Engl J Med. 2017;377:936–46.
22. Varricchi G, Bagnasco D, Borriello F, et al. Interleukin-5 pathway inhibition in the treatment of eosinophilic respiratory disorders: evidence and unmet needs. Curr Opin Allergy Clin Immunol. 2016;16:186–200.
23. Magnan A, Bourdin A, Prazma CM, et al. Treatment response with mepolizumab in severe eosinophilic asthma patients with previous omalizumab treatment. Allergy. 2016;71:1335–44.
24. Kelly EA, Esnault S, Liu LY, et al. Mepolizumab attenuates airway eosinophil numbers, but not their functional phenotype in asthma. Am J Respir Crit Care Med. 2017;196:1385–95.

25. Mukherjee M, Aleman Paramo F, Kjarsgaard M, et al. Weight-adjusted intravenous reslizumab in severe asthma with inadequate response to fixed-dose subcutaneous mepolizumab. Am J Respir Crit Care Med. 2018;197(1):38–46.
26. Laviolette M, Gossage DL, Gauvreau G, et al. Effects of benralizumab on airway eosinophils in asthmatic patients with sputum eosinophilia. J Allergy Clin Immunol. 2013;132:1086–1096.e5.
27. Ferguson GT, FitzGerald JM, Bleecker ER, et al. Benralizumab for patients with mild to moderate, persistent asthma (BISE): a randomised, double-blind, placebo-controlled, phase 3 trial. Lancet Respir Med. 2017;5:568–76.
28. Vatrella A, Fabozzi I, Calabrese C, et al. Dupilumab: a novel treatment for asthma. J Asthma Allergy. 2014;7:123–30.
29. McCormick SM, Heller NM. Commentary: IL-4 and IL-13 receptors and signaling. Cytokine. 2015;75:38–50.
30. Gonem S, Berair R, Singapuri A, et al. Fevipiprant, a prostaglandin D2 receptor 2 antagonist, in patients with persistent eosinophilic asthma: a single-centre, randomised, double-blind, parallel-group, placebo-controlled trial. Lancet Respir Med. 2016;4:699–707.
31. Bateman ED, Guerreros AG, Brockhaus F, et al. Fevipiprant, an oral prostaglandin DP2 receptor (CRTh2) antagonist, in allergic asthma uncontrolled on low-dose inhaled corticosteroids. Eur Respir J. 2017;50:1700670.
32. Gibson PG, Yang IA, Upham JW, et al. Effect of azithromycin on asthma exacerbations and quality of life in adults with persistent uncontrolled asthma (AMAZES): a randomised, double-blind, placebo-controlled trial. Lancet. 2017;390:659–68.

MIX
Papier aus verantwortungsvollen Quellen
Paper from responsible sources
FSC® C105338

If you have any concerns about our products,
you can contact us on
ProductSafety@springernature.com

In case Publisher is established outside the EU,
the EU authorized representative is:
Springer Nature Customer Service Center GmbH
Europaplatz 3, 69115 Heidelberg, Germany

Printed by Libri Plureos GmbH
in Hamburg, Germany